AGING
BACKWARDS

AGING BACKWARDS

UPDATED AND REVISED EDITION

REVERSE THE AGING PROCESS
AND LOOK 10 YEARS YOUNGER
IN 30 MINUTES A DAY

MIRANDA
ESMONDE-WHITE

HARPER WAVE
An Imprint of HarperCollins*Publishers*

Learn more about how to age backwards and download
free videos of the workouts featured in this book by visiting:
www.essentrics.com/agingbackwards.html.

AGING BACKWARDS: UPDATED AND REVISED EDITION. Copyright © 2018 by Miranda Esmonde-White. All rights reserved. Printed in the United States of America. No part of this book may be used or reproduced in any manner whatsoever without written permission except in the case of brief quotations embodied in critical articles and reviews. For information, address HarperCollins Publishers, 195 Broadway, New York, NY 10007.

HarperCollins books may be purchased for educational, business, or sales promotional use. For information, please e-mail the Special Markets Department at SPsales@harpercollins.com.

FIRST EDITION

Designed by Kris Tobiassen of Matchbook Digital
Exercise photographs by Jessica Blaine Smith

Library of Congress Cataloging-in-Publication Data

Esmonde-White, Miranda.
  Aging backwards : reverse the aging process and look 10 years younger in 30 minutes a day / Miranda Esmonde-White.
      pages   cm
   ISBN 978-0-06-231333-1 (hardback)
  1. Rejuvenation. 2. Longevity. 3. Aging—Prevention. 4. Physical fitness.   I. Title.
  RA776.75.E66 2014
  613.2—dc23

                                                                            2014028452

ISBN 978-0-06-285932-7

    19   20   21   22   ov/lsc   10 9 8 7 6 5 4

CONTENTS

PART III: THE EIGHT AGE-REVERSING WORKOUTS

THE MYTH OF AGING

Every day, no matter what our age or current health status, we have a very clear choice: We can grow older or we can grow younger.

I mean this quite literally.

Some people might not see aging as a choice—they see it as something they have no control over, just like the passage of time. But with the information I share in this book, I hope to convince you that you absolutely *do* have a choice in the age of your bones, your muscles, your internal organs, and your skin. You can decide if you want to spend your days feeling vital, energetic, and healthy, and joyfully use your body to exercise, travel, and play with your children (or grandchildren)—or if you want to be confined to a life of joint and back pain, limited mobility, and a lack of physical strength that keep you sitting on a bench and watching others do the things you once did.

The difference between these two extremes is a matter of 30 minutes a day—that's all. You already possess the power to determine your body's true age. The choice is yours: Passively allow the aging process to take over, or actively counter the aging process in a mere half hour a day.

Me, I like that kind of deal. I plan on staying young forever (or as close to it as I can manage!). And I hope you do, too. I can show you how.

THE MYTH OF AGING

Until very recently, medical researchers believed that many of the negative effects of aging were inevitable. As we grow old, conventional wisdom has told us, our skin sags, our muscles waste away, we gain weight, and we eventually develop a chronic disease, such as heart disease or cancer, which will kill us. (Is it any wonder we are such a youth-obsessed culture?)

But in the past few years, scientists have made tremendous discoveries that offer a different picture of what it looks like to get older. Consider these common myths about aging that have recently been disproved:

Myth: Our brains grow only until we're in our twenties—and then they start to die.

Truth: Neuroscientists have proved that, as long as we stay mentally active, our brains can actually keep growing and adding brain cells well into our twilight years, through the miracle of "brain plasticity." (And the most powerful booster of brain plasticity? Exercise.)

Myth: Our metabolism slows down when we hit 40.

Truth: If we do absolutely no exercise, yes, our metabolism will start to take a hit at 40. But study after study over the last 25 years has proved that people who consistently exercise three times a week can completely avoid age-related metabolic slowdown and actually retain the same metabolism as people almost 40 years younger.[1–3]

Myth: Our skin will inevitably age and wrinkle—our only defense is good genes.

Truth: We know now that many, many factors have an impact on the health of our skin. And, luckily, the amount of sun exposure can be countered with sunscreen. The amount of free radical activity can be countered with a fruit- and vegetable-rich diet packed with free radical–fighting antioxidants. The impact of gravity on the skin's elasticity and firmness can be lessened with plenty of fresh water, enough deep sleep, and—you guessed it—exercise. (Recent research found just 3 months of exercising twice a week can restore the skin of 60-year-old sedentary folks to the same state as that of a 20- to 40-year-old!)[4]

Myth: Our muscles inevitably fade away with each passing decade.

Truth: If we don't use it, we will lose it. But if we *do* use it—meaning, if we engage our muscles—we don't need to lose a single ounce of muscle. One University of Pittsburgh study looked at a cross section of 40 recreational athletes aged 40 to 81 who exercised four or five times a week. They underwent MRI scans, body composition testing, and quadriceps strength testing; the researchers measured their muscle mass and the amount of fat under their skin and between their muscles. The researchers found that, with exercise, the athletes could retain exactly the same levels of lean muscle mass from their forties into their eighties—in fact, some of the older exercisers had even more lean muscle tissue than the younger athletes.[5]

Myth: Our joints are destined to fail.

Truth: Our joints fail not from age but from mismanagement. If we learn how to protect our body from intense impact (by learning to walk gently), pay attention to range of motion in our training, and learn the proper ways to support our joints with flexible muscles, our original joints—the ones we are born with!—should remain healthy until our very last days.

Myth: Everyone gets cancer/diabetes/heart disease eventually.

Truth: Up to 34 percent of cancer risk is directly attributable to lifestyle choices.[6] Every kilogram of weight loss lowers your risk of type 2 diabetes by 16 percent—so losing just 10 pounds could reduce your diabetes risk by *over 60 percent*.[7] A study in the *New England Journal of Medicine* estimated that 82 percent of heart disease and heart attacks in women can be attributed to factors such as smoking, not exercising, being overweight, or eating a high-glycemic-index diet.[8]

If these truths seem hard to believe, I'm not surprised. The dogma has long held that we are powerless against the march of time. After all, research had long found that, between the ages of 40 and 50, adults lose up to 8 percent of our muscle mass, with the loss accelerating to over 15 percent per decade after we hit 75.[9] The assumption has always been that this muscle loss was simply an inevitable consequence of aging.

But just in the last five years, the field of aging research has exploded with new clinical findings. Those scientists from the University of Pittsburgh and other well-respected medical centers have been proving just how wrong the assumption that age equals muscle loss has been. They've found that aging is far more a consequence of lifestyle choices than of calendar years. In fact, many of the symptoms we associate with aging are actually the result of not just the wear and tear on our bodies from years of use but also the negative effects of *disuse*. In our muscles are the keys to our longevity—the mystical wellspring of youth, called the mitochondria—the powerhouses of the cells. If we can keep these mitochondrial fires burning, our muscles—not to mention our bones, hearts, lungs, skin—can all enjoy the vitality and energy of youth, right up until our final days.

The secret to keeping these powerhouses well fed and burning strong may surprise you. You don't have to run marathons. (Unless you want to.) You don't have to spend hours grunting in the gym. (Unless you're into that kind of thing.) All you have to do is something that takes just a few minutes every day and makes your body feel lighter, leaner, smoother, more graceful, and relaxed. All you need to do is *stretch*.

LOSE 10 POUNDS AND 10 YEARS IN 10 MINUTES

Now, I'm not talking about the kind of stretching you do as you get out of bed and yawn in the morning. When I say stretching, I'm referring to a very specific kind of stretching, the ESSENTRICS model of toning and strengthening, which I will share with you in this book. Throughout my 30+ years of creating, developing, and teaching this approach, I have seen how it helps people instantly improve their appearance and very quickly improve many aspects of their health and fitness. I've been amazed at how the ESSENTRICS model can radically change the lives of busy people who thought their fittest years were behind them. And I love to see the looks on people's faces when they realize how quickly good posture can radically change their appearance. (As I like to say, by using the ESSENTRICS model, you can "lose 10 pounds and 10 years in 10 minutes"— simply by changing the way you carry your body, you will look a decade younger.)

In working with thousands of people on every continent in the world, I have seen how the ESSENTRICS model:

- improves core strength
- lengthens and tones all muscles (for a "dancer's body")
- increases energy, balance, and flexibility
- speeds lymphatic drainage and circulation

- improves circulation and cardiovascular tone

- decreases the need for prescription drugs

- relieves back, knee, shoulder, hip, and foot pain

- rebalances joints; alleviates and reverses arthritis and osteoporosis

- heals acute and chronic injuries

- decreases falls, sprains, and other injuries that can lead to inactivity and lack of mobility

and, most delightfully for many,

- helps speed weight loss—without extra effort

All of these remarkable benefits can be yours for just the slightest investment of time every day. If one drug could offer all of these benefits, we'd be beating down our doctors' doors for prescriptions, and the pharmaceutical companies would be rich beyond their dreams. We all have access to these benefits—and many more—every day. Give yourself just 30 minutes, and very soon, you will be leading a better, richer, longer, healthier, and happier life. Not a bad trade!

I have taught this method to Olympic athletes, arthritic retirees, busy working parents, aspiring actors and dancers—and even professional hockey players. All these diverse groups of people have been surprised by how pleasurable, simple, and quick exercises can make such a profound difference in their lives. This simple approach has been a life-changer for thousands of people—but the very first life it changed was my own.

THE DANCE OF LIFE

The idea of the ESSENTRICS model was born when I was just a girl, studying at the National Ballet School of Canada, and then in my work as a professional ballerina with the National Ballet Company. There I developed a combination of discipline and creativity (not to mention an intimate knowledge of form and physique) that sparked my imagination for research and exploration, but I wouldn't develop the techniques until much later. I had to understand the need first.

After dancing in one too many *Nutcracker* performances, I left the company and started my own company, then was lured into the corporate world. I enjoyed the glamorous but grueling travel schedule, which had me leaving my 5-year-old daughter with relatives two weeks a month. Leaving that job was the best decision I ever made, though at the time it seemed like the most irresponsible. I had no job, and had no inkling as to how I was going to support my little Sahra as a single mom.

I started teaching fitness classes at a local church to make ends meet. With strong word of mouth, my aerobics classes rapidly gained popularity, and before I knew it, I was teaching almost five classes a day in the basement of a church. I was outgrowing the space, and decided to dream big and open my own fitness center. As I began to discuss my work with more and more people both within and outside the fitness community, I came to realize that most people really didn't love to exercise. The members of my studio enjoyed my classes, sure—but I gradually became aware of this huge number of people who weren't walking in my door and didn't do any exercise, at any time.

This fascinated me—why did they not enjoy something that gave me so much pleasure and satisfaction? I surveyed many non-exercisers to find out, and what was revealed to me was the fact that people actually *did* want to exercise—they just didn't like what was being offered. While aerobics had taken the fitness world by storm, we heard plenty of complaints about it, too. For many, the loud pounding music, high-impact movements, and copious sweating, and the bulky muscle tone they seemed to develop, were all strong deterrents. I kept hearing from my members, especially the women: *I would like a workout with smooth movements that stretches me out instead of bulking me up. I want to have a long, lean, slender body.* In other words, a dancer's body.

Well, I could certainly help with that! I set out to create an "anti-aerobic" workout. With thorough research and the invaluable mentorship of the director of Oncology and Surgery at Montreal's Royal Victoria Hospital, Dr. Shibata, and a retired sports physiotherapist, Fiona Gilmore, I dived deep into the subjects of anatomy, physiology, and basic kinesiology. As the owner of the center, I had the ability to offer trial classes to a select group of students who guided me into designing a program that was fun, was healing, and, most important, slimmed them down and toned their bodies in the ways that they hoped exercise would.

What came out of these classes was the foundation of the ESSENTRICS approach, a method I called the Esmonde Technique, which forms the basis for this book and for all the other fitness programs I have ever developed. All of these classes were aimed at keeping participants young and healthy, from cradle to grave.

I named my first class Classical Stretch because the workouts stretched the muscles with long, simple, elegant lines that reminded me of classical architecture. When I opened Classical Stretch classes to the public at my fitness center, they were an instant hit. They became so popular that, to fill the demand, I had to train new instructors to teach my technique.

Having to train others forced me to get my method out of my head and onto paper, to make it teachable to others. I had to dissect the technique and figure out what it was before I could train anyone else. I spent much of that time with my nose in any medical, anatomical, and physiological manuals I could get my hands on. This marked the beginning of a 10-year process of writing my own manuals, testing them, and starting again. I went through that process three times before completing a series of four manuals, levels one to four, which are the basis of our teacher-training program.

After experiencing surprisingly huge growth in the program, in 1999, I worked up my courage and approached PBS with the faint hope that it might be interested in airing my fitness program on its network. Well, the rest is history. Fifteen years later, *Classical Stretch* is still viewable daily in millions of U.S. households. Thousands of Americans wake up to do the program daily.

Over the years, we've worked to create better descriptions for this powerful method, so we can do a better job of training people. Many have said they think of ESSENTRICS as a flexibility program, with a bit of tai chi, some elements of physiotherapy stretching, and a lengthening of the muscles similar to that of ballet. When we named our program Classical Stretch, we were confident that it was a flexibility program, since everyone who did it gained flexibility.

But here's the thing: We kept receiving testimonials from viewers of the TV show and from our own clients telling us about the dramatic changes in their strength, weight, and body shape. If they stuck with it, people found ESSENTRICS would elongate their legs, hips, and stomach, not to mention their arms, neck, and shoulders; improve their posture; slenderize their shoulders; lengthen the pectorals and upper back; open the chest and elongate the neckline; reduce love handles; and eliminate underarm flab. After a few weeks of intense ESSENTRICS, they weren't the only ones noticing these changes—they found a measuring tape and a camera helped them see startling changes in the length and shape of their muscles. Many lost a pants size, or more.

We were baffled. We didn't think it made sense that stretching was causing these changes in strength, weight, and body shape. Even though we knew that people were losing weight while doing the program, we couldn't figure out why. In our search to identify what Classical Stretch was, we ended up finding the answer in the science of movement and muscle anatomy. We had our epiphany.

According to sports science, you can strengthen your muscles in one of two ways: eccentrically or concentrically. Concentric exercises strengthen the muscle by shortening it; eccentric exercise strengthens the muscle by lengthening it.

Most other fitness programs focus on concentric strengthening. You see concentric strengthening every day in the gym, when people tense up and shorten their quadriceps muscles as they attempt to straighten a leg on the leg extension machine, for example, or pull a hand weight toward a shoulder in a biceps curl, or "crunch" their abdominal muscles during a sit-up. That concentric motion is typically where we focus all of our workout attention—we don't give as much attention to lengthening our muscles.

But by ignoring this, we're giving short shrift to a very critical aspect of the development of healthy, strong muscles—eccentric exercise. Eccentric exercise simultaneously lengthens and strengthens, and is just as critical as concentric exercise, but is often overlooked as "wasted" time. In fact, your body is actually doing eccentric exercises as you reach into a high cupboard or get out of a car: You bend a knee and stretch out your quadriceps while these are still bearing the full weight of your body as you stand up. You are strengthening while lengthening.

Just as in the physics maxim, "The longer the lever, the heavier the load," eccentric exercise allows your "lever" (muscle) to easily bear more resistance while in its lengthened position. The result: simultaneously lengthened and strengthened muscles.

Once we realized eccentric exercise was the principle at work in Classical Stretch, suddenly we understood why people were losing weight while following our program. Muscle cells burn more calories, so when you increase the difficulty of the load on the longer muscle, you increase the mass of your muscle, you increase your body's metabolic rate, you burn more calories, and you lose weight. At this point, we didn't realize something even more amazing about eccentric exercise—something that wouldn't be revealed for years, something that helped us to understand what it is about ESSENTRICS that makes it such a powerful antiaging program. As the scientific community began to shed new light on how our DNA ages, we learned that eccentric exercise specifically, directly, and powerfully communicates with our cells to reduce oxidative stress on a cellular level—in other words, to directly combat aging.[10] And this powerful weight loss and antiaging component, eccentric exercise, was in virtually every minute of every Classical Stretch routine.

Even after we solved the mystery, our ideas took a while to catch on. Instructors had never come across a workout based on eccentric strengthening, and the results people were finding in our program flew in the face of many theories they had been taught to believe. In fitness circles, the idea that flexibility could increase strength and help in weight loss seemed absurd. But as skeptical as our colleagues in the fitness industry were, we continued to receive an overwhelming number of weight loss testimonials from viewers and students around the world. Classical Stretch—now known as ESSENTRICS—was clearly a very powerful technique for both weight loss and strengthening.

In addition to fitness-seekers' stunning weight loss, we have continued to see good results in many other groups of people as well, everyone from new mothers to baby boomers to retirees, giving us endless proof that the ESSENTRICS method increases flexibility; rebalances joints; relieves back, knee, shoulder, hip, and foot pain; and does much more for a wide spectrum of people. We see it heal injuries and alleviate and reverse arthritis and osteoporosis. We see it straighten out severely rounded backs and give participants wonderful posture. We are thrilled when it helps athletes win Olympic medals and championships. All along this journey, we have seen countless people following Classical Stretch or doing ESSENTRICS who easily lost weight and shed inches in their so-called problem areas, making their body shape longer and leaner—all of this from a method that can be done in as little as 30 minutes a day. This is the kind of full-body transformation that I would like to share with you.

AGE BACKWARDS, STARTING TODAY

I know you are busy, juggling a full schedule of competing responsibilities in your work and in your life. The ESSENTRICS method helps you maximize your exercise time investment by helping you achieve all of your strength, flexibility, balance, agility, and weight loss goals simultaneously. In this book, I will explain exactly how and why the ESSENTRICS approach is so powerful and how you can use it to slow down and reverse your own aging process.

In Part I, "How and Why We Age," we'll talk about the startling physical changes that can pop up around our forties, some of which can suddenly make us feel "old," and how we can respond to fight them. I'll reveal how mitochondria of our cells hold the keys to many facets of our health, and how dozens of recent studies suggest we need to change the way we look at aging. In Part II, "How We Stay Young and Healthy," I'll discuss all the benefits of the ESSENTRICS approach and how it works to keep us young, limber, and disease-free. In Part III, "The Eight Age-Reversing Workouts," I'll share easy-to-follow 30-minute workouts for specific conditions and goals, including losing weight, relieving pain, increasing balance, and reversing osteoporosis and arthritis. In each of the workouts, you'll see me; my daughter, Sahra; and James Gadon, an ESSENTRICS instructor, in step-by-step photos with clear descriptions that explain the finer points of each exercise. I will explain how the ESSENTRICS technique not only reconnects you with your body's innate strength and grace on a daily basis but also reconnects you with the joyful pleasure of movement in every aspect of your life, increasing your energy, smoothing and firming your skin, and bringing a sparkle back into your eyes.

I'm in my sixties—over forty years have passed since I danced *Swan Lake*—but I still feel great! I am pain-free, energetic, and strong. I have a spring in my step and I look forward to every new day with happy enthusiasm. When I get sick, I recover rapidly. I really value being full of energy and leading a pain-free life. I know how I have achieved this gift, and I want to share how you, too, can easily achieve it.

Whether you are a 40-year-old working parent needing a quick home-based workout, a 50-year-old executive who needs to de-stress and rebalance between meetings, or a 65-year-old who is looking for new ways to stay fit and vital, I hope that *Aging Backwards* provides you with the inspiration and understanding to feel and look stronger, healthier, and happier—for many years to come.

Enjoy!
Miranda

PART I

HOW AND WHY WE AGE

CHAPTER 1

WHAT IS AGING?

Your body wants to move.

Your body was designed to stay strong, vital, and pain-free for the full duration of your life, no matter how old you get.

Your body was programmed with the ability to continually repair itself after damage. Whether your living machine is mending broken bones, torn muscles, cuts, and burns, or fighting off invading forces with its immunity soldier cells, its primary objective is to heal. And the more you move, the more you fuel this amazing cellular regeneration and these positive, adaptive responses to challenges.

Yes, your body was created with complex systems that are capable of keeping you active and vibrant well into your senior years. And the sharpest, most powerful, most versatile tool for retaining this radiant ageless youth is not your heart, or your brain, or your lungs—it is your muscles.

Your muscles have an innate ability to remain strong and flexible well into old age—a function that not only helps you feel and move better but also helps every single body system function better. When your muscles are strong, you

- feel less pain

- have better circulation

- lower your blood sugar

- increase your energy

- enjoy better focus, stronger memory, and sharper thinking

- grow significantly more brain cells

- bring more oxygen into your body

- lower your cholesterol

- improve your cardiovascular health

- slash your risk of diabetes, cancer, Alzheimer's disease, high blood pressure, and other chronic diseases

- become more flexible, limber, and mobile

- easily maintain a healthy weight and a toned physique

Muscles can do all that for you, and more. Even when people come to exercise late in life, and even if they have previously been completely sedentary, miraculous turnarounds are possible. I have watched in awe as people in their forties, fifties, sixties, and even seventies who do just a bit of exercise every day enjoy their ability to run a road race, hike mountain trails, go for (and get!) a challenging new promotion at work, or even just twirl their children or grandchildren around in the air.

What unites all these people is an understanding that if you use your muscles, you'll never have to lose your muscles—you can retain all the vigor, energy, strength, and vitality of youth indefinitely. And you can get the bulk of these benefits with just a little bit of exercise—only 30 minutes—per day.

Working with the ESSENTRICS system, I've helped thousands of people learn an approach to exercise that's exactly the opposite of the unproductive, dangerous "no pain, no gain" philosophy of yore. In fact, in contrast, I'd say ESSENTRICS is the "no pain, all pleasure" school of fitness. Using my program, you can strengthen your muscles, protect your body against chronic disease, gain tremendous energy, and get to enjoy a long and lean "dancer's body" to boot—all in the time it takes you to watch one episode of a television show.

And let's not forget the ultimate reward: You'll live longer.

A recent longitudinal study analyzed data from more than 650,000 people whose medical information had been recorded for 10 years. Among the astonishing findings the researchers reported was the fact that for every minute you exercise, you lengthen your life by 7 minutes. These effects were found among people who started exercising at 45 years old for just 150 minutes a week—the same as doing the ESSENTRICS program five times a week. And that was just the start; those who exercised more often had even greater results.[11]

A guaranteed 1-to-7 return on your investment—that's an astounding ratio. You can't beat that kind of return in any stock market. Isn't that amazing? You don't have to be an athlete or a professional dancer and you don't have to win the genetic lottery to reap these kinds of health rewards. You just need to stretch—following a very specific, scientifically validated approach—for about a half hour a day. But before we learn about the program itself, let's dig a little deeper to find out why the muscles are so important in protecting and optimizing the health of everyone's system, and how we can capitalize on their versatile powers right away.

YOUR GENES ARE NOT YOUR DESTINY

Before I started exploring the subject of aging, I believed that loss of muscle mass and decrease in energy were controlled by chronological years. I always thought it was a matter of good luck or good genes that enabled some people to stay youthful and active as they aged while others did not. In fact, genes have very little to do with it. Research suggests that only 25 percent of our longevity is determined by our genes—the rest, 75 percent, is due to lifestyle and environmental factors.[12] And one of the most impactful of these factors is—no surprise here—exercise, adding as much as 8 extra years to our lives. Our bones, our cardiovascular system, even our skin—every one of our body systems can stay strong and vital for the duration of our lives, simply through the miracle of a daily dose of modest stretching exercise.

We haven't always known this elementary fact. Many of us have had a brush with death at some time in our lives, because of either an illness such as cancer or heart disease, or, in some cases, a serious accident. We saw the brittle bones, the stoop, the shuffling walk as simply being part of growing old. Yes, it could be argued that those symptoms were "normal" and "natural"; what we were seeing was the body's natural process of deconditioning and muscle deterioration. But the fact that a process is natural doesn't necessarily mean it is *inevitable*.

Consider the options open to any gardener: If she tends to her garden, diligently watering her plants and ensuring they get the right amounts of sun, nutrients, and water, her plants will flourish and grow. If, however, she neglects her garden, it will soon become overgrown with weeds and, without nutrition or water, the plants will die.

Both of these outcomes are equally "natural." These are two choices with two different consequences, both following the laws of nature. But no one would argue that they are equally desirable. Many people used to allow their bodies to age prematurely simply because they did not know any better. Do you remember how surprising it used to be, about twenty years ago, to see an elderly person with good posture and vitality, a senior who lived without chronic pain or any health problems? In the not-so-distant past, those people were seen as unusual and extraordinary.

Now, we see many people who are examples of radiant health at 60, 70, even 80 and 90 years old. We see 93-year-old yoga teachers, academics making scientific discoveries into their eighties, heads of state governing until their late eighties. We see Betty White, still cracking people up and delighting audiences at 92. We are finally starting to understand that we hold most of the power of healthy aging in our own hands.

So what does lifelong vitality look like? Many people wonder what their life would look like if they were to invest the time to do the ESSENTRICS program. I tell them this:

You *can* maintain perfect posture for life. Perfect posture is more natural than a slouched back, as the body is designed to have and to function with perfect posture. Slouching is caused by a disintegration of the musculature through lack of use. Slouching is the human equivalent of a plant being choked by surrounding weeds, causing the muscle cells to die before their time. But good posture is the most natural and healthy state for the spine. The muscles of the torso are created to be strong and mobile. If we take care of our spinal muscles, our posture will remain vertical, and the functioning of all of our internal organs will benefit.

You *can* continue to be limber and move with energy and vigor for life. Having a spring in our step is the way the body is designed to walk. The muscles of the feet, ankles, knees, and hips are created to be strong enough to easily power a light, relaxed walking gait. Neglect of those muscles causes them to shrink and weaken, but just a bit of gentle exercise will keep them strong and dynamic. If you do walk with this kind if lightness and agility, you will be less likely to suffer from any aches, pains, and stiffness, and you will feel young even as you get older. Most aches and pains are the result of stiff, atrophied muscles, and these problems, left untreated, will only worsen as we age. The truth is that there is absolutely no need for the majority of muscular-related chronic aches and pains to occur in the first place. If we exercise our muscles with an equal emphasis on strength and flexibility, they will give us a spring in our step that will last throughout our lives.

You *can* stay slim and toned for life. Uncontrollable weight gain may seem like a side effect of aging, but it's entirely avoidable if we do the correct flexibility and strengthening exercises. Weak, inflexible muscles make us look soft and shapeless, and those unnecessary body changes rob us of our self-esteem and confidence. True, we might not be running down the beach in a bikini forever. But who really wants that? We can easily retain a trim waist and narrow hips, even build muscle definition, and radically reduce the dreaded "softening" in our midsections through regular gentle full-body stretching and strengthening exercises.

OK, I've made my point: The rapid decline of the human body is not an inevitability that must be accepted and endured—we now know it's something that doesn't have to happen at all. But the question for many of us is: How do we prevent that from happening? What do we do about it?

WHERE TO GO FROM HERE

You might have a regular exercise routine—but still struggle with chronic pain that derails your program regularly. Or you may be losing weight through diet, but you aren't sure about what kind of exercise you should be doing. Or you may have gone all out on an ambitious exercise program—only to burn out, get discouraged, and fall into a habit of inactivity, waiting for the next thing that will inspire you into action.

Simply put, many people are stuck in neutral, not knowing where to begin. We may see the marathon runners or the spin class junkies, and we know that's not for us—but how do we get started? Is it more important to focus on strength training or cardio? Should we work out for a long time at a low intensity, or for a short time at a high intensity? We might put off starting a program until a not-so-busy time. We may spend time debating which program would be better than another. We may wander around in the bookstore or fitness equipment aisle, and wonder, "Which one of these do I do?"

Anytime I hear people asking these questions, I can't wait to share ESSENTRICS with them. Because I know that in this one program, they can fulfill so many of their health and fitness goals. No matter if you're already in great shape, or if you've just getting back on the exercise horse, or if you've never been active a day in your life, the same program works for everyone. Here's why:

- You can do it anywhere—at any location, inside or outside, where you have one body length of space, you have enough room.

- You need no equipment—you can exercise in your pajamas, and you don't even need fancy shoes. (In fact, ESSENTRICS should be done barefoot!)

- You don't need a lot of time—the entire program can be completed in 30 minutes or less.

- You don't need to be super fit—the ESSENTRICS program is progressive, starting gently and becoming more challenging to your muscles as you go.

- You won't ever feel "pain"—the ESSENTRICS program is relaxing and all about limbering up and stretching all of your muscles as you strengthen them.

- You can lose weight without sweating—one amazing feature of ESSENTRICS is how powerfully it can shape your physique, helping you develop stronger muscles that burn fat while you sleep.

All that is required to feel youthful and healthy is a little bit of help from doing this daily gentle full-body exercise. You may be surprised to know that something so gentle can be so beneficial, because we've been told that exercise must hurt—we have to go for the burn if we're going to see any results. But many people dislike rigorous exercise. The truth is this: To remain strong and flexible, we do not have to push our bodies to their limits. Even modest exercise will grant an exponential return in value.

If you have always resisted the idea of exercising, you probably tried exercises that are uncomfortable, unnatural, and exhausting. The truth is that exercising should feel natural, and the ESSENTRICS program will show you how 30 minutes of exercise can be fun and pleasant. You'll learn how to *enjoy* exercise again, and even look forward to your next session. If you're already a practiced exerciser, you'll be surprised and delighted to find a stretching, strengthening, lengthening, and toning method that leaves you feeling so relaxed and limber while it also gives you such amazing results in only 30 minutes a day. I believe that ESSENTRICS will completely change your perspective on exercise.

PROTECT YOUR LEGACY

Once you understand how your body ages, you will see that you absolutely *do* have a choice about how you live the rest of your life. One choice: Do nothing, and just allow yourself to slow down, get stiff, suffer chronic pain, and most likely lose your independence. Another choice: Stay young, vibrant, energetic, and independent. In this book, my goal is to share everything you need to make the choice to keep your body vital and engaged in the world for as long as you choose. By the end of this book, you will learn, beyond a doubt, that that choice is entirely in your hands.

Helping everyone, especially older adults, learn to love exercise isn't just my profession—it's my mission. From a societal perspective, I believe we too often dwell on what we lose as we age instead of focusing on what we gain. I firmly believe we should *never* conceal our age—as though having lived all of our exciting years is something that we should be ashamed of! What we need to do is realize that, every day, we can be walking, living, breathing examples of lives well lived. We need to safeguard our health with exercise not only for the sake of our vanity but also to share our knowledge and protect our legacy. After all, the beauty of aging is that by the time we've hit our "second half," we have become wiser, better people with a wealth of maturity and life experience. We learn to tolerate others' perspectives, values, and outlooks. We may even come to celebrate these differences! Perhaps most important, we learn to forgive, and come to understand what is truly worthy of our time and focus, and what is not. Just when we are emotionally ready to make the world a better place and help guide the younger generation, our aging bodies can sometimes get in the way.

What a shame it would be if all of your accumulated knowledge, gleaned from a lifetime of hard lessons learned, could be wasted because your body is not vital enough to stay in the game.

Let's not let that happen. The world needs your wisdom.

You *can* make a different choice. You can choose to live a life full of vitality, strength, and joy. Whether you are a fitness lover or a casual walker, or even if you've never exercised a day in your life, you can make that happen—you just have to start *now*!

The first step toward realizing the importance of your choices is to understand *why* some bodies begin the steady decline of age—and how, instead, you can protect your lifestyle, your brain, and your gorgeous body by learning to *Age Backwards*.

CHAPTER 2

THE BUILDING BLOCKS OF LIFE AND OUR INNER FOUNTAIN OF YOUTH

A full understanding of successful aging must begin with the primary building blocks of your body: your cells.

You are the sum of trillions of cells. The health and vitality of your cells are reflected in every single tissue in your body. Whether you can run and jump, or feel compelled to sing or laugh, whether you enjoy a calm and peaceful afternoon with friends, or stand on the podium in a room full of your peers to deliver a speech, the health of your cells determines how your body will respond to each of these activities. If your cells are well nourished and stimulated, your body's natural response will be energetic; you will manage stress well; your blood pressure and blood sugar will be balanced; and you'll stay physically youthful and vibrant. If your cells are not well fed and not well stimulated, they begin to atrophy and die, and you can start to feel sluggish, depressed, and in pain.

With all of your trillions of cells, you might be tempted to brush off the significance of some cell loss—you've got more where those came from, right? But when it comes to *Aging Backwards*, every single cell counts—you don't want to allow any harm to come to a single one of them.

Among your body's brilliantly and intricately arranged cells, there are various types: brain cells, nerve cells, blood cells, hair cells, egg cells, sperm cells—more than 200 major types of cells in total. All of these cells work in unison to keep one another and your entire system alive, healthy, and functioning—and there are many ways you can help them do just that. Before we learn how to keep them alive and thriving as long as possible, let's first review a bit about cells and their function, so we can gain a full appreciation of how important it is to support their work, especially the work of the powerful and mighty mitochondria.

ANATOMY OF A CELL

Our cells are responsible for our every biological function, and they all share a few distinct characteristics. Each cell is surrounded by a cell membrane, inside of which you'll find cytoplasm. To get a sense of the structure of a cell, think of a balloon filled with thick jelly. That balloon, the cell membrane, is made up of protein and fat, and it cautiously guards the materials inside the cell. Only certain things are allowed into and out of the cell—primarily, food goes in, waste comes out.

Inside the cell, the cytoplasm is made up of fatty acids, sugars, enzymes, and amino acids, all components that help the cell do its work. The nucleus is the mastermind of the cell, housing our DNA, the master genetic code. The nucleus keeps busy by controlling the cell's food intake, movement, and reproduction. Cells contain several other important parts, called organelles, each with its own function. The kind of organelle that is our chief ally in the defense against cellular aging is the dynamic, ever-changing powerhouse, the mitochondria.

MIGHTY MITOCHONDRIA

Every single cell requires a source of energy to power its life. This energy "power plant" is called a mitochondrion. Most cells have only a small number of mitochondria, but muscle cells have so many—in the tens of thousands—that scientists have not yet been able to count them all. The reason muscle cells hold the key to staying younger is that they house 95 percent of the body's mitochondria. In recent years, scientists have discovered that not only do mitochondria power the cells; they also play a huge role in our rate of aging and the length of our lives. Mitochondria can keep us young—as long as we protect and nurture them.

Mitochondria are the digestive system of our cells. They take in nutrients, break them down using enzymes and oxygen, and then create energy for every body part to use to fulfill its assigned task. This process of generating energy, called "cellular respiration," creates adenosine triphosphate (ATP), an energy-transfer molecule. When a cell needs energy, the mitochondria convert carbohydrates (in the form of glycogen) or fat into energy and then ATP shuttles the energy to whatever part of the cell needs it. Almost every bodily function that requires energy gets it via ATP. While the amount of ATP in our body remains relatively stable, this stockpile of ATP operates like a battery: We use up the power and then we replenish it, with help from our mitochondria. Mitochondria are one of the most primitive parts of the cell—they may have originated as free-living single-celled organisms. They even have their own mini set of DNA, which can be affected by our lifestyle choices, just like the DNA in the cell's nucleus.[13]

With every move we make, we communicate directly with our mitochondria. Movement activates the mitochondria, turning them "on," and a sedentary lifestyle deactivates them and turns them "off." When we move our muscles or exercise, we actually increase the quantity of mitochondria, and this increase in turn gives us more energy to burn. But when we allow our muscles to become weak, we have fewer mitochondria, so we have less energy and fewer calorie-burning furnaces to keep us slim.

People who are fit usually have a lot of energy, because their mitochondria are powered up and ready. By contrast, less fit people have a smaller supply of mitochondria that is barely sufficient to fulfill limited physical needs. As a result, they may have difficulty with basic tasks like walking up and down stairs, getting out of a chair, or even getting out of bed.

This is the honest truth: The only difference between strong people and weaker people lies in what they demand of their muscles. *Anyone* can have strong muscles because, by definition, muscles are created to be strong and they can be made stronger with very little time or effort.

Our bodies want to move. Our body's natural state is to be packed with strong, energy-producing, fat-burning muscles.

MITOCHONDRIA FUEL ALL CELLS

Muscles control all of our body movements, whether voluntary or involuntary. In addition to the skeletal muscles that we control voluntarily, such as our arm, leg, and back muscles, we have other muscles over which we have no control, working 24 hours a day. These involuntary muscles include the cardiac or "heart" muscle, as well as the smooth muscles of our blood vessels, bladder, and digestive tract. These muscles continue working nonstop every day of our lives, performing tasks essential to life, including maintaining a rhythmic heartbeat and controlling our breathing. Even when we're not exercising, every muscle in the body requires mitochondria to keep operating. So over and above the calories our muscles use during activity, the entire body requires energy to fulfill these day-to-day functions, serving all the systems of the body, such as the nervous system, digestive system, and skeletal system. We need a fixed amount of calories just to keep our trillions of bodily cells cared for and each of these cell's mitochondria fueled. Even before we get out of bed in the morning, the calorie-burning, energy-producing factories are working away, and then regular exercise can stimulate these furnaces to burn even more calories.

Do you need a bit of a motivational boost to stick with your exercise program? I like to picture my mitochondria as calorie-burning factories, and just knowing that 95 percent of these "factories" are found in my muscles motivates me to use my body more often. Or I envision my mitochondria as the fire underneath the cauldron of my metabolism—every step I take adds a piece of wood to the fire that's "cooking" my excess pounds and keeping me slender.

We create more and more mitochondria every time we walk to the corner store instead of driving, every time we take the stairs instead of the elevator, and every time we park farther away from, not closer to, the door of a mall or shopping center. Try to think of your mitochondria as you pull your own suitcases through the airport, as you garden, or as you push the vacuum to do your own housecleaning. Every single one of these opportunities concentrates the power of your energy-producing mitochondria.

The more you move on a regular basis, the more energy you demand from your mitochondria, and the more alive and fired up they will be. When you run up and down stairs on a regular basis, you constantly demand that your existing mitochondria supply you with lots of energy. Repeat this often enough, and your muscle cells compensate by creating more mitochondria, so that everyday tasks become easy and effortless. Someone who regularly challenges her body will not be likely to get even the slightest bit tired running up and down stairs. But someone who never runs up and down stairs, whose body is unaccustomed to the strains of regular exercise, will have fewer mitochondria supplying energy and will therefore find this task very tiring.

When people don't exercise on a regular basis, any strenuous effort rapidly drains their few available mitochondria, zapping their energy and leaving their muscles sore and depleted. Their deconditioned lungs don't have enough oxygen, and they feel winded. Their deconditioned heart feels overtaxed, and it might be racing. They may even be sweating from the effort. They would be likely to find themselves completely exhausted and incapable of doing more exercise or physical activity until the cells were replenished, a recovery period that could take several minutes.

However, if these people persisted in running up and down stairs every day for a few days, their mitochondria would multiply, their muscles would strengthen, and they would rapidly find the task much easier to perform.

The human body is remarkably resilient. We are designed to be strong and able to do things like run up the stairs with ease. That's why, with relatively little effort and time, your muscles happily and eagerly strengthen, quickly making a task that was once a challenge an absolute breeze.

The energy-producing benefits of mitochondria are obvious and immediate. But for many people who've struggled with cutting calories and portions to lose weight, mitochondria's ability to speed weight loss is also a huge plus.

MITOCHONDRIA REGULATE OUR WEIGHT

To explain the relationship between mitochondria and weight loss, I often think of my body as a home furnace. Let's say I decided to have a lazy day and not turn my mito-chondria furnace on. The furnace would just sit there, inactive, not burning any of my calorie fuel, and the tank would remain full. If I then continued to order more fuel, the tank would fill up, running out of room. In order to complete the delivery, the fuel oil company would have to leave the extra fuel in storage tanks around my house. To reduce this unnecessary surplus around my home (and around my hips!), I'd have to turn my mitochondrial furnace on and burn the excess fuel, as well as go on a fuel "diet" and reduce my future orders from the company to ensure that I get only as much fuel as I need and no more.

We do not need extra tanks of fuel hanging around our waistline. We do need to keep a balance, make an effort to burn what we consume, and not consume more food than we can burn. But even more than that, we need a furnace that's burning bright, torching those calories 24 hours a day.

If burning calories during exercise were the only weight management feature of exercise, you would find it virtually impossible to exercise enough to keep your weight under control. To give you an idea of how difficult it would be to rely solely on exercise as a means of burning calories, consider this case:

Take a 150-pound person who runs for a half hour, moving at 10 miles per hour; she would burn approximately 600 calories. If she ate an 8-ounce steak (approximately 500 calories) and a 7-ounce baked potato (approximately 250 calories), her run would not be sufficient to burn all of the calories from even that small meal. She would have to run much, much more in one day to burn through her normal consumption of thousands of calories—sometimes almost two hours a day.

Clearly, the idea of using exercise to counterbalance an overconsumption of calories is not going to work—you'd be facing an uphill road. If you want to keep a steady weight, you need to keep a clear head when it comes to consumption and manage portion sizes. As the saying goes, "You can't exercise away a bad diet."

BELLY, HIPS, AND THIGHS— ENEMIES OR BEST FRIENDS OF WEIGHT LOSS?

One irony about weight loss is that among your body's greatest allies are your belly, hips, and thighs, the very body parts many women bemoan during their efforts to shed pounds. But the muscle groups in these areas and along our spinal column are the largest such groups in our bodies. The larger the muscle groups, the more mitochondria they contain, so the more we exercise our large muscles, the more calories we will burn. (Check out Chapter 11 for some simple weight loss exercises to help increase your calorie-burning rate by using these major muscle groups.)

But the calorie-burning function of exercise actually does have an important role in weight loss. **The primary role of exercise in weight loss is the prevention of cellular atrophy or death.** Mitochondria loss after age 40 is the beginning of the unexplained weight gain that we tend to call "age-related" slowing down of the metabolism. But this metabolic slowdown has less to do with age than it has to do with a lack of activity—and a stubborn refusal to change habits!

Many of us tend to eat the same portions throughout life. But when you enter old age without exercising regularly or adjusting your caloric intake, two things happen: Your muscle cells atrophy or die through lack of use, leaving you with fewer mitochondria than you had when you were younger; and your unchanged portions run smack into your greatly changed ability to burn them. Result: unwanted weight gain that steadily increases every year.

You don't need to feel helpless to fight a flagging metabolism. Understanding the relationship between cells, mitochondria, and regular exercise is the key to controlling your weight while empowering yourself to stay young forever. Let's dig a little deeper into how our bodies age, and how our choices can play a major role in slowing, stopping, or even reversing the primary causes of metabolic sluggishness and physical aging.

CHAPTER 3

"WHY DO I SUDDENLY FEEL SO OLD?"

HOW YOUR BODY RESPONDS TO THE BIG 4-0

Many people dread turning 40. While there's nothing to fear if you do take care of yourself, the cold hard truth is that if you don't, two things begin to happen around this time: cell death and atrophy. These natural processes are not inevitable—we have ways of fighting back, and those ways are not at all difficult. You just have to learn what's happening within your cells, so you can understand how to stop this process and turn back the clock.

THE LIFE SPAN OF A CELL

We begin our lives as cells with the union of a sperm and an egg, setting off a frantic but efficient multiplication of cells as they form our bones, heart, eyes, skin, and every other body part. All of those trillions of muscle, brain, nerve, and blood cells participate in this frenzy of cell division that takes us through the various stages of development, from fetus to infant to toddler to adolescent and, finally, to a mature adult.

Throughout this time, cells don't just spring into being and live indefinitely, of course. New cells are created and old cells die in a constant state of cell turnover. Cells are preprogrammed for apoptosis, or planned cell death, and they wait for a signal—from either inside or outside the cell—to initiate their own death. During development, apoptosis is the body's way of building itself according to our genetic blueprint, acting as a sculptor's knife to carve out our distinct features, such as our fingers and toes. Apoptosis is also what helps us learn new information and preserve our memory by pruning out unused neurons and decluttering the brain. Between ages 8 and 14, we lose 30 billion to 40 billion cells a day and constantly generate new ones.

Once we hit adulthood, and our growth process is completed, a new process of repair and replacement begins. Apoptosis steps up the pace and causes between 50 billion and 70 billion of our cells to die every day, just to maintain homeostasis and balance out the new cells being formed.[14, 15] This process continues for approximately two decades, until we are about 40, when we enter the next stage of life, and the repair and replacement process becomes a little unwieldy because, by that point, our cells have divided so many times. Each time they divide, in the process of copying their DNA, cells take a snip off our telomeres, the protective caps at the end of our 46 chromosomes. Once they've divided about 50 times, the telomeres are almost gone, and they send a stern message to the body to stop cell division. The cell heeds the call, essentially sending out an emergency message similar to what happens when the DNA is damaged by dangerous radiation or chemicals.[16] That's when we exit the repair and replacement stage, and enter what's known as "cellular senescence" (from the Latin word *senex*, meaning old age or old man),[17] which I refer to as "cell death."

Every living thing follows a similar life pattern, consisting of a period of growth and maturity, a period of stabilization, and, finally, a slow period of decomposition and decay. Whether it is a plant, an animal, or a human being, every living thing follows a natural cycle of life to death. But just as the nature of our gardener's tending can make her flowers either enjoy a long blooming period or wilt prematurely, there are certain things we can do to hasten this process, or slow it down, or potentially even reverse it.

For decades, scientists have debated various theories about how aging affects the body. Some believe that accumulated oxidation damages our cells and that this oxidation is the primary culprit. Oxidation occurs when free radicals produced by cellular respiration—or taken in via environmental exposure to, for example, secondhand smoke, pesticides, and pollutants—cause our cells to lose electrons. The result is destructive; just think of what happens to iron when it is oxidized—it rusts. The thinking goes that if enough of the molecules in our cells, including our DNA, are damaged, the process of apoptosis may go a little haywire.[18] At that point, our body hits a tipping point, our tissues and organs start to deteriorate, and disease takes root.[19]

Recently, scientists have begun to home in on this same process taking place within the DNA of mitochondria. Many are now saying that mitochondrial function is the true key to unlock the mystery of aging, and it is the decrease in the number and the health of our mitochondria that determines how aging affects health.[20] Another new strain of research has found a link between the two theories on aging, suggesting that our mitochondria actually communicate with our cells' telomeres, telling them whether they should shorten, and thus hasten aging; or not shorten, helping to slow down or stall the aging process.[21]

The research is still evolving and I expect we will gain even more valuable insights into the aging process in the next few years. But in the meantime, it would appear to be in our best interest to befriend and care for these very influential little power plants. So what can we do to make sure we have plenty of healthy mitochondria to give our telomeres the message to stay long indefinitely?

Our genetics do play a role here—but not the leading role. Perhaps you're blessed with long-lived parents and grandparents. Even so, don't bank on living long yourself without some intervention. Experts believe that only 30 percent of our longevity is determined by our genes. If we've inherited genes that make us more susceptible to cancer or heart disease, we can't exchange those for new ones. But what we absolutely *can* do is take care to protect ourselves from the worst of those genetic messages. The growing field of "epigenetics"—which studies everything that happens to your genes *after* the moment you're born—tells us that certain behaviors switch on positive genes and switch off negative genes, or vice versa. The choices we make during our lifetime determine the level of "burden" on our bodies. The more healthy choices we make, the lower our genetic burden, and the lower our chances of genetic harm. (One maxim of epigenetics is "Our genes load the gun, but our environment pulls the trigger.")

Even if we live "clean," we are all living in a modern and sometimes toxic world and, over the course of our lives, we encounter a certain amount of environmental challenge to the health of our DNA. This damage to each person's genome accumulates with time, and the risk of mutation increases every time a cell divides and its DNA is copied. We can have the greatest impact on how those genes are expressed by controlling the environment in which they are expressed, shielding our cells from environmental assaults: excess radiation from the sun, stress, poor nutrition, chemicals, lack of sleep, and dozens of other factors that cause oxidative stress and that have been proved to damage us genetically.[22]

But in addition to playing defense, we also have a very powerful offense on our side: eccentric exercise.

Eccentric exercise, the type that defines the ESSENTRICS method, has been shown in animal studies to directly communicate with the mitochondria in our cells to reduce oxidative stress on a cellular level—in other words, to directly combat aging.[23]

Another specific agent in our bodies helps to protect our telomeres by improving mitochondrial function to stop those messages of destruction: an enzyme known as telo-merase.[24] And what has been proved to increase telomerase, as well as protect telomeres, prevent mitochondria loss, and stop cell death—all effects that can help lengthen our life span and improve the quality of our lives as we grow older? Exercise.[25–29]

Have you started to notice changes in your body—a loss of energy, unexplained weight gain, poor posture, or changes in body shape? These changes reflect the messages that your cells and your DNA have been receiving for years. But the choices you make in your daily life, starting today, can put the brakes on these messages and help stall the triggers for cell death. Act now and you can truly begin *Aging Backwards*.

AGING SNEAKS UP ON US

The progress of our life cycle is barely perceptible to us on a day-to-day basis because changes are happening at the cellular level, one cell at a time. We see it only in retrospect, when we compare what our lives were once like with what they've become. Children have this realization more often—they know they're maturing when they are suddenly able to do activities that they were previously incapable of doing, such as riding a bike, raiding the high cupboards for cookies, or playing certain sports. These milestones are tangible proof that allow a child to become aware of his or her own growth and maturation.

On the other side, as we hit the window of change after repair and replacement, it's the things we can *no longer* do that become the milestones we notice. We might find it more difficult to run to catch a bus, or we may lose the ability to play certain sports. Or we may even find it difficult to do everyday tasks that we had no trouble doing beforehand, such as opening jar lids or carrying heavy groceries in from the car. We notice changes in our energy level when activities we did with ease last summer, such as mowing the lawn or gardening for hours, have become an exhausting chore this summer. Perhaps the starkest realization comes when last year's clothes don't fit anymore!

Because this process is so slow, we barely notice it happening. We see it only when we compare photos of ourselves over the decades and see the changes in our shape and weight, and notice new wrinkles. We are blissfully unaware, on a daily basis, that we are fading slowly, one cell death at a time—and thank goodness for that! Who wants to be reminded of aging every day? But this slow fading does us no favors—sometimes those stark realizations can be just what we need to stay vigilant if we're to prevent premature aging. Let's take a closer look at what is going on here, at the cellular level, so we can gain the awareness that can spur us to action.

THE FIRST RISK: THE TRANSITION FROM CELL REPAIR TO CELL DEATH

At around age 40, and with every passing decade after 40, the message not to repair or replace dead cells becomes more aggressive. In our early forties, that message is weak, but it gains momentum quickly. The cellular decline is mirrored by a similar downshifting in other physical systems. Women's estrogen levels and men's testosterone levels decline. Especially if we don't exercise much, our heart and lungs become weaker. Our balance becomes less steady. Our blood vessels collect more calcification, restricting the free flow of blood throughout the body. Each of these negative developments influences others in turn, and the cumulative effect can be dramatic. Most of us have witnessed the aging of parents, friends, and grandparents and are astounded by their rapid deterioration in their seventies or eighties, or even sooner—but experiencing it ourselves is a whole different matter.

While we have made huge strides in medicine over the past few decades, the fact of the matter is that scientists have not definitively connected all of the dots—they still don't know exactly how to stay young and prevent cell loss. When I started looking at the cells as the basis of life and growth, I really wanted to know two things: (1) What triggers the maintenance of cells? (2) What causes this maintenance phase to end? Specifically, I wanted to know if we could prolong the repair and replacement phase, and delay or even block the message that allows for cell death.

We can get a general idea of people's ages just by observing the posture or energy levels of randomly chosen adults. People in their twenties usually have more energy, are stronger, and stand up straighter than 60- or 70-year-olds. When you compare a young adult with an older one, the physical differences are obvious. Something has changed to cause these outward signs of aging—what is it?

As we've discussed, from the moment we are born there is a continuous turnover of cells in the body as new cells are created to replace damaged and dead cells. From childhood through young adulthood, the message to repair and replace dying and damaged cells is issued automatically, but that message wanes as we age. In order to turn off the maintenance message, something new must happen, something to signal a change. That "something new" must be more than just chronological aging—otherwise it wouldn't vary so much from person to person. In order to keep the "repair and replace" command in effect instead of allowing the "let die" command to take over, we have to somehow *prove* to our body the necessity of these cells.

We know that the message to atrophy gets transmitted to muscle cells only when they are not being used. So it follows that the way to put the brakes on the cell death process is to send the message loud and clear: "I still need these muscles! I'm still using them!" And the only way to do that, to prevent any message of atrophy to reach any part of your body, is to use each and every one of your 620 muscles *each and every day*.

If you're accustomed to regular exercise, you've probably intuitively felt this all along: As long as you are using a muscle, its cells will continue to be repaired and replaced. We see this knowledge at work in the medical, surgical, and physiotherapy communities. Hospital patients, for example, are encouraged to get out of bed and begin moving as soon as the doctor tells them it is OK to do so, which is often only hours after an operation. As torturous to the patient as getting up may seem, doctors know the serious consequences of remaining sedentary following surgery. Exercising after surgery is intended to prevent muscles from shrinking and atrophying, which would render full recovery much slower and less successful. This principle applies even more compellingly when you begin in a state of relatively good health, and especially robust health.

In 2011, the University of Pittsburgh conducted a study of muscle atrophy and chronological aging. The researchers looked at cross sections of muscle tissue of 40 high-level recreational athletes who were 40 to 81 years old and trained four or five times a week. After analyzing their body composition and quadriceps strength, and taking an MRI of their quadriceps, the researchers found something that rocked the medical field:

The lean muscle tissue of a 74-year-old triathlete was essentially *equal* to the lean muscle tissue of a 40-year-old who worked out just as often. The study debunked previously accepted theories, the "common knowledge" that decline in muscle mass and strength was a natural part of aging. Instead, the researchers had definitive proof that muscle cell loss was a consequence of inactivity, and not of age.[30]

These findings are applicable to others as well as athletes. Statistics show that the average person who does a minimum amount of daily exercise, and has a somewhat sedentary, somewhat active lifestyle, loses an average of 7 to 8 percent of her body's cells every decade. On the other hand, an active person who performs regular exercise using the entirety of her musculature loses an average of only 2 to 3 percent of her cells each decade. This is such a vast improvement that by age 60, the more sedentary person will have lost up to 25 percent of her muscle cells, compared with an approximately 8 percent loss in the active person.

ESSENTRICS can help you achieve these results faster than any other program, because eccentric exercise is the most efficient and effective form of muscle training. A Swiss study of people with heart disease between ages 40 and 66 found that, after 8 weeks on a program to compare the impact of concentric versus eccentric training, those who'd followed the eccentric program could produce *four times* as much power as those who'd followed the concentric program, despite having a similar feeling of exer-

MUSCLE MASS REMAINING PER DECADE

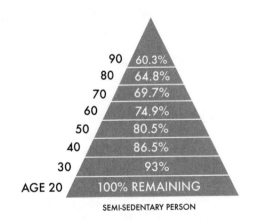

90 60.3%
80 64.8%
70 69.7%
60 74.9%
50 80.5%
40 86.5%
30 93%
AGE 20 100% REMAINING

SEMI-SEDENTARY PERSON

7% of muscle mass loss every decade for a semi-sedentary person.

Note that by age 60, a semi-sedentary person would have approximately 75% of muscle mass remaining, reducing energy level and dramatically changing the shape of the body.

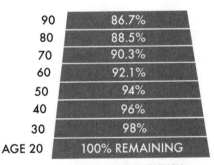

90 86.7%
80 88.5%
70 90.3%
60 92.1%
50 94%
40 96%
30 98%
AGE 20 100% REMAINING

PHYSICALLY ACTIVE PERSON

2% of muscle loss every decade for a physically active person.

Note that by age 60, a physically active person has approximately 92% of muscle mass remaining, which would mean that the person has lots of energy and the body has not changed shape very much.

tion. In other words, for the same effort, the eccentric exercisers got four times the benefit. And, significantly, their blood pressure and various other measures of cardiac stress were not raised at all. For heart patients, this indicates a safer form of exercise while they recover from a dangerous cardiac event. For the rest of us, it simply means we can get stronger, more flexible, and leaner, and look younger—all without spending hours on the treadmill and possibly without even having to break a sweat![31]

I've seen this effect firsthand dozens of times, even in my own family. When my mother was celebrating her eighty-ninth birthday, I brought her to Mexico to join a one-week group fitness holiday. Each day began and ended with a one-hour fitness class. The first day she sat through the classes doing the exercises in her chair. The second day, she did the standing exercises for 15 minutes and then sat down to do the rest of the exercises. By the third day, she was doing 30 minutes of the class standing, and by the end of the week she was doing one complete class a day. After the fitness holiday, she

ARE YOU SEDENTARY?

A lot of people think that if they work out once a day, they're "active"—even if they sit at a desk all day. Not true. Studies show that sitting too much is literally deadly. A recent National Health and Nutrition Examination survey of about 5,000 people found that between 50 and 70 percent spent 6 or more hours sitting every day.[32] When sitting is combined with commuting, eating, sleeping, and other stationary activities, other estimates put our sit/lie down total at closer to 21 hours a day.[33] You may be watching TV for hours a day or working hard at your desk, but your body doesn't know the difference. When you sit for most of the day, you face the same degree of risks from chronic debilitating diseases as a habitual smoker. (Researchers call sedentary behavior "the sitting disease" and even say that "sitting is the new smoking.")

Take every opportunity to stand—while reading a memo, talking on the phone, having a meeting. (Better yet, do a walking meeting!) Set a timer on your phone to remind you to stand up every half hour—just getting some blood flow through your legs will help combat some of the risks. Even better would be to get a standing desk, so you can do your work and stand up at the same time.

returned home reenergized and feeling like a different person, with enough energy to work in her garden and visit friends as she thoroughly enjoyed a new outlook on life.

Perhaps even more dramatic is the effect ESSENTRICS can have on younger people who have been active but have slipped out of the habit of regular exercise. I have a friend with a demanding desk job who spent hours sitting every day. When I shared some of the research on the health risks of sitting too long, she started doing ESSENTRICS every morning and also bought a standing desk. With her computer and her phone at her desk, she went from sitting for 8 to 9 hours a day to sitting 6 to 7 hours a day and doing 30 minutes of exercise in the morning. Those two little changes helped her to lose more than 20 pounds and lower her blood sugar and cholesterol in a matter of months. She now does her ESSENTRICS every morning, walks at lunchtime, and is looking forward to running her first 5K. And she looks about 10 years younger.

We are never too old to feel young! Over the years I have seen scenarios similar to my mother's and my friend's hundreds of times, as people revitalize their lives with full-body, gentle, and regular exercise. Nothing feels as good as feeling young in your own body.

THE SECOND RISK: ATROPHY

Now we know a bit more about cell death, which was previously considered "normal aging." We now can clearly see that movement and activity are very powerful means of forestalling cell death. But cell death is not the only way that our bodies lose their cells. Another way is atrophy.

Atrophy is a very slow process through which a healthy cell gradually shrinks until it shrivels into extinction. Any shrinking of the cells impairs the functioning of your powerful furnaces, the mitochondria. Instead of actively working, tens of thousands of mitochondria shrink and disappear along with the cells. The more your cells atrophy, the more mitochondria disappear.

Atrophy can happen at any age to anyone, from children to seniors. In most cases, it can be slowed down and reversed if it is caught early enough. But why does it happen? In one word: immobility!

Muscles can become immobilized in many different ways—not only through disuse but also through overdevelopment. (I'll explain more about this in Chapter 6.) In other words, atrophy can happen to people who are in shape as well as those who are out of shape or those who are simply sedentary.

The best example I can give to clarify the power of immobility is a broken bone locked for several weeks in a cast. When the cast is finally removed, the once-broken limb is visibly shrunken and weaker than the corresponding, undamaged limb. It is at this point that a doctor will encourage the patient to undergo a physical rehabilitation program designed to stimulate the atrophied cells to rebuild and strengthen weakened muscles.

Broken bones and forced confinement in plaster casts are not the only ways that muscles can become immobilized; they are merely the most extreme and familiar example. A sedentary lifestyle—too much time spent on couches or at desks and not enough movement—is the most common trigger for muscular atrophy. When we move our muscles as little as possible, with a sedentary lifestyle, we turn down our furnaces and literally cause our muscles to atrophy. When the cells atrophy, we feel even more tired because we have fewer mitochondria generating ATP. A vicious circle begins: less energy leading to less movement, which leads to less energy, which leads to less movement.

Atrophy from a sedentary lifestyle leads to weight gain, loss of energy, and chronic aches and pains. But atrophy can be easily prevented, stopped, and even reversed with daily gentle full-body exercise. The start of reversing atrophy is the same as preventing cell death: We have to turn on our mitochondria in order to restore our cells to full working order. Daily exercise "reboots" the shrunken cells, reversing atrophy and supplying sufficient energy to make exercising easier. With very little exertion, you can experience a positive change in your energy and strength almost immediately. When people aren't accustomed to exercising, even basic movements can feel difficult. This difficulty can lead to a negative attitude toward fitness, making recovery even more challenging. It is a slippery slope: The less you do, the more challenging exercise becomes, robbing you of your motivation. This consistent disuse triggers cell atrophy in the first place, but don't be discouraged. Early-stage atrophy is easy to reverse. Your body has strong regenerative powers; it wants to move and will reward you for movement.

Physiotherapists describe the three stages of muscle atrophy in the following way:

- **Stage one** occurs when people can move their muscles under their own steam but it is really difficult and exhausting.

- **Stage two** is reached when these people are no longer able to move their muscles by themselves because their muscles have become too weak. However, with the assistance of someone else doing the actual manipulation, the muscles are somewhat pliable.

- **Stage three** is reached when the cells have totally atrophied; at that stage, the muscles are rock solid and totally immovable. In stage three, it is essentially game over for the atrophied muscles: the damage is irreversible.

If you have noticed that your energy level is lower than it used to be, that your weight and body shape are changing and seem to be more difficult to control, or that you suffer from chronic aches and pains, you are experiencing early symptoms of cell atrophy! Many people wait until they notice these changes before they consider addressing the problem, but ideally we want to prevent these symptoms before they set in and affect your life. But once these symptoms do set in, it is crucial to make changes—if you don't do anything, each of these problems is only going to worsen, compounding your troubles and accelerating the aging process.

Although atrophy can happen to anyone at any age, you can see it most often among people who are starting to age, beginning around age 40. Some other signs of atrophy include:

- poor posture
- rounded back
- stiff movements
- walking slowly
- restricted range of motion
- tension or stiffness in your gait
- stiffness in hips, spine, or legs
- trouble getting into and out of a car
- trouble walking up and down stairs

We want to avoid stage 3 atrophy at all costs, and reverse any stage 1 or stage 2 atrophy that has already begun. In my years as a personal trainer, I have seen many people in their seventies reverse stage 2 atrophy, usually in the upper back. It requires daily exercise and persistence, but the rewards are well worth the effort. Atrophy is commonly reflected in poor posture, which can create a host of other issues associated with aging.

If you spend time people-watching, you will see signs of atrophy everywhere: not just in the limp of an aging woman with an ache in her hip, but in the slight hunch

ARE YOU AT RISK?

While neurogenic atrophy tends to occur suddenly or severely, when a nerve that connects to a muscle is injured (as in a broken bone) or diseased (as in ALS), the atrophy we're talking about here comes about mainly through a lack of physical activity over a specific time period. Those most at risk of atrophy that occurs as a result of disuse are:

- people with sedentary jobs requiring them to sit at a desk all day
- people with medical conditions that limit movement
- people who've been bedridden for a few days or longer
- people whose decreased activity has corresponded with a "shrunken" appearance

Symptoms of atrophy include:

- "wasting" appearance, when lean muscle tissue seems thinner and less substantial than previously
- curved back, indicating onset of sarcopenia or osteoporosis
- shuffling gait or limp

Thankfully, disuse atrophy can be reversed with good nutrition and exercise. Atrophy is the most literal visual definition of "move it or lose it."

of a marathon runner or the spinal stiffness of a former basketball player. I hate seeing how widespread these problems are, and it pains me to point them out to people, but I know what these symptoms lead to and how debilitating and painful they become if left untreated. Atrophy begets more atrophy, and as one muscle group becomes stiff and immobile, its neighboring muscle groups will experience the same problems. This creates a dangerous chain reaction that is best addressed sooner rather than later.

At a certain point, it becomes hard to tell the difference between cell death and atrophy. Cell death is something that must be prevented to be overcome. We must act now and continue the fight as long as we possibly can.

THE PERILS OF GOING OVERBOARD

All movement is preferable to no movement, but a variety of movements are far better than just a few movements. Some of us are obsessed with finding just one form of exercise and sticking with it. But in order to send the message "I'm still here!" loud and clear, the best approach for your body is to do many different types of movements, so you can hit all of your 620 muscles. Choosing to exercise only certain parts of the body, with the vague hope that the other muscles will get strengthened through some form of osmosis, will have negative ramifications—sometimes among the "fittest" people we know.

Many popular fitness programs and sporting activities target primary muscles, using exercises or machines that rely on repetitive, robotic movements. They also contract muscles to strengthen them. This concentric exercise results in compression and shorter muscle fibers, as well as pain, injury, and lack of mobility. Instructors and clients alike mistakenly believe that an injury or pain is due to the fact that the clients are getting old. The truth is that these well-intentioned people have been unknowingly damaged by the very training they were doing to stay healthy!

To keep all 620 muscles from aging, you have to honestly assess all the different ways you exercise. I certainly don't want to deter you from any specific exercise or sport that you love. I just ask that you make sure to find time to move your less commonly used muscles at some point every day. Even some of the most popular exercises—such as walking, sit-ups, and weight machine work—can affect your muscles in ways you wouldn't expect.

Walking is fun, a social activity that gets us out in the fresh air, but it engages primarily the leg muscles, meaning that the torso and upper body are largely neglected. If walking were your only source of exercise, some 300 upper body muscles would be allowed to age and atrophy! ESSENTRICS can be a nice complement to a daily walk to help engage the muscles above the waist.

Sit-ups are the most well known of the basic core exercises, done with all kinds of fancy machines or simply by lying on the floor. Sit-ups engage mostly the front of your trunk, strengthening your abdominal muscles. Even when done correctly, all forms of sit-ups engage only about 100 muscles.

Most people don't do sit-ups correctly; they often use the head as a pump to help lift the shoulders off the floor. This causes neck pain and does nothing for the actual abdominal muscles that sit-ups are intended to strengthen. Sit-ups can also lead to all kinds of spinal injuries, especially when modifications for an individual's shape and body type are not taken into consideration. Perhaps the most disheartening problem for those who do sit-ups is that, when done incorrectly, they can result in a very strong, round muscle mass around the stomach—exactly the opposite of the desired flat abdominal muscles.

The ESSENTRICS core program featured on page 129 will help you strengthen as you lengthen, so that you develop a stronger core and back muscles to ensure the proper posture and the flatter stomach you've been hoping for.

Most exercise equipment or machinery offers opportunities for strengthening targeted muscle groups. These exercises are concentric, which means that they shorten or contract the muscles in strengthening them. After years and years of contracting or shortening, the muscles will begin to squeeze the joints, restricting movement and range of motion, and leading to stiffness, pain, and arthritis.

In addition to the long-term problems brought on by shortening of the muscles, most fitness equipment is not designed to work through the full range of motion of any joint; instead it isolates and strengthens specific individual muscles. The result is muscular imbalance, as some muscles are strengthened while adjoining muscles remain weak, which inevitably leads to discomfort and possible injury. These machines limit the number of muscles they recruit, leaving hundreds of others untouched. (And as we now know, unused muscles in people over 40 are destined to atrophy and die!)

Some of the worst posture I have ever seen is in people who overdo upper body strengthening. They're so focused on increasing how many pounds they can lift that they fail to notice the damage they're doing to their back muscles as they overtrain the upper body. Certainly the most bizarre form of atrophy I've seen is in weight-lifting enthusiasts who have overbuilt their muscles to the extent that these muscles have become immobile. If you take a close look at bodybuilders (or people who aspire to be like them), you will see not just impressive biceps but also rounded backs and poor posture.

When I work with these people, I find that they also have very limited movement, flexibility, and range of motion in their muscles. They come to me when they approach 40 and are in pain due to the extreme contracting of their muscles. The atrophy from having permanently contracted muscles is excruciating.

In our instructor training for ESSENTRICS, I've worked with former yoga, Pilates, weight-lifting, and aerobics instructors. Most of these fitness experts are suffering from various degrees of atrophy caused by repetitive pounding, pumping, or holding a pose or position for extended periods of time. They are shocked when they see what has happened to their own muscles because their fitness programs typically train body parts (such as the abs and butt), but they've never trained the whole body as a unit. How upsetting that the people who are most dedicated to doing the right thing for their bodies and their clients' bodies unwittingly cause them damage! They put so much effort toward staying healthy and in shape, and yet the focus on strengthening without flexibility makes their muscles unhealthy.

As greater numbers of high-performance athletes and everyday "weekend warriors" grow older, the signs of atrophy caused by overtightening the muscles will become more obvious. The first symptom is pain, which is likely to be followed by chronic injuries—the result of 10 to 15 years of intense training with minimal flexibility work to counteract the tightening of the muscles. The impact on the joints and muscles from years of playing squash, tennis, or football; running; or extreme weight training first shows up as bulky, rigid muscles. Many athletes don't know how to maintain a balance between strength, flexibility, and range of motion, perhaps not appreciating that range of motion is just as important as strength, not only for performance but to prevent injury. Often, the athletes who were admired as gods or goddesses in their youth are riddled with pain and discomfort in their late thirties and early forties, requiring hip or knee replacement surgery, or regular cortisone injections to loosen rigid muscles.

Sadly, thousands of once fit individuals are aging prematurely because they've been injured by incorrect training. We have all heard stories of a favorite athlete whose body is destroyed before age 50. Such athletes are experiencing a form of muscle atrophy, one that can be prevented or reversed with corrective flexibility exercises to release the tension causing the immobility and pain. Reversing this type of atrophy is difficult, however, and requires a lot of patience. It can take months, even years, to completely reverse the damage caused by strengthening the muscles without paying equal attention to range of motion or flexibility.

THE PERILS OF DOING TOO LITTLE

As dangerous as it is to overtrain and overspecialize, it is far more common not to exercise enough. To me, the situation is most tragic when a person has developed disdain for exercise and avoids it at all costs. Some people have had a bad experience in a high school gym class, have tried programs that were too advanced, have shied away from the often prohibitively high cost of gym membership, or simply feel they do not have the time for daily exercise.

People cite many reasons why they don't enjoy exercising. I'm going to try to help you overcome all of those reasons by showing you that doing gentle, full-body exercise for 20 to 30 minutes is actually enjoyable. A good exercise program is one that not only challenges your body but also is well suited to your fitness level. A good exercise program is one that you will actually look forward to doing because it feels good *while you are doing it*. And a good exercise program is one that will also give you real results you can see and feel throughout the rest of your day.

It is never too late to slow down and reverse the aging process. Now you know that aging is caused by cell atrophy and cell loss and that it can be prevented, slowed down, or reversed with exercise. Now is the time to fight for your youth!

EVERY MUSCLE COUNTS

There is no cheating when it comes to preventing the negative effects of aging; our muscles know when they are and aren't being used. When we fail to engage all 620 muscles of our body, the message to "let die" will slip out from those fallow muscles and start spreading throughout your body. After the age of 40, people who are inactive, overly sedentary, or simply doing the wrong exercises are signaling to their master control that they do not need their muscles, triggering the message "Let the cells die."

In addition to these global triggers of decomposition, the individual muscles we don't use will atrophy and lead to an unbalanced body that results in pain and injury—which will only further accelerate aging. Unfortunately, the body's master control doesn't give any free passes!

The ESSENTRICS technique is quite simple and easy to do, and was designed to engage all 620 muscles with exercises that mimic daily life. By using each and every muscle, you are sending a message to your body every day: "Hey, I still need that one!" Full-body exercise is the secret to preventing cell death. Let's learn more about how engaging each one of those muscles acts as a megaphone to our DNA, shouting loud and clear, "I want to live!"

CHAPTER 4

MEET YOUR MUSCLES, LIGAMENTS, JOINTS, AND FASCIA

We've talked about how essential it is to move your muscles and why we need to move all 650 of them on a regular basis. To understand how this applies to the method behind ESSENTRICS, we need to stop thinking about each muscle as an individual unit. Instead we need to start thinking of our muscles and joints as a complex, interlocking system that relays communication throughout our bodies, on a second-by-second basis, via a massive network of connective tissue.

Since I wrote this book in 2014, an incredible amount of research has been conducted on this topic. Researchers have investigated what exactly connective tissue is, how it works, and why its optimal functioning is so critical to our health as we age. Every day, studies from around the world add more insight to our understanding of this integral, yet largely unknown, part of our biology. We're learning that many of the symptoms of aging—stiffness, poor posture, reduced mobility, a limited range of motion—actually have their root in connective tissue problems.

Connective tissue interacts with all other tissues in the body to such a degree that some scientists now believe it might be a "meta-system": a communication network that integrates all the body's mechanical forces and influences the function of our physiological systems. Some experts believe connective tissue may even be a "missing link" in medicine, key in helping us understand why a physical injury or illness in one part of the body may cause a cascade of effects in other distant, seemingly unrelated areas of the body.[34] (It may even explain the concrete physiological underpinnings of the 2,000-year-old discipline of traditional Chinese medicine, such as the theorized existence of energy meridians and their influence on the movement of *chi*, or "life force," in the body.) If these theories are true—and I believe they are—it's absolutely clear why keeping our connective tissue supple, resilient, and injury-free is a critical part of safeguarding this communication system, thereby helping our entire body remain healthy, youthful, and vibrant as we age.

CONNECTIVE TISSUES AND THEIR FUNCTIONS

Ligaments: Attach bone to bone, have little or no ability to repair themselves if torn or overstretched

Tendons: Connect muscle to bone, have minimal elasticity, heal slowly

Cartilage: Provides a frictionless surface; cushions and prevents wear on joints

Fascia: Fibrous material that covers, surrounds, separates, and joins bones and muscles; suspends our organs

Extracellular Matrix ("Oily Bath"): Watery substance within connective tissue that nourishes and permits ease of movement for muscles

FASCIA: THE TIES THAT BIND

Imagine a collagen-rich, stretchy slipcover for every organ, nerve, bone, and muscle in our bodies, and you start to get a sense of how fundamental connective tissue—specifically fascia—is to the entire body. Suspending our organs inside our torso, connecting our head to our back to our feet, fascia protects, supports, and literally binds our body together. Fascia can be gossamer-thin and translucent, like a spider web, or thick and tough like rope. Ounce for ounce, fascia is stronger than steel. Other specialized types of connective tissue include bones, ligaments, tendons, cartilage, and fat (adipose) tissue. Even blood, strictly speaking, is considered connective tissue. But to me, the most exciting aspect of the latest research on connective tissue relates to fascia.

Fascia is the stretchy tissue that forms an uninterrupted, three-dimensional web within our body. Our body has sheets, bags, and strings of fascia of varying thickness and size, some superficial and some deep. Fascia envelops both individual microscopic muscle filaments as well as whole muscle groups, such as the trapezius, pectorals, and quadriceps. For example, one of the largest fascia configurations in the body is known as the "trousers," a massive sheet of fascia that crosses over the knees and ends near the waist, giving the appearance of short leggings. This fascia trouser is thicker around the knees and thinner as it continues up the legs and over the hips, thickening again near the waist. When the fascia trouser is healthy, supple, and resilient, it acts like a girdle, giving the body a firm shape.

Fascia helps muscles transmit their force so we can convert that force into movement. The system of fascia is bound by tensile links (think of the structure of a geodesic dome, like the one at Epcot in Disney World), with space and fluid between the links that can help absorb external pressure and more evenly distribute force across the fascial structure. This allows our bodies to withstand tremendous force instead of absorbing it in one local area, which would lead to increased pain and injury.

Fascia is also a second nervous system in and of itself, with almost 10 times the number of sensory nerve endings as muscle. Helene Langevin, director of the Osher Center for Integrative Medicine at Harvard Medical School, has done landmark studies on the function and importance of connective tissue and its impact on pain. One of the leading researchers in the field today, Langevin describes fascia as a "living matrix" whose health is essential to our well-being.

When I first studied anatomy textbooks, there were no illustrations or photographs of these filmy, slippery membranes or the irregular lobular wraps of connective tissue woven throughout the human form. As I learn more from contemporary research, I've started to rethink my entire approach to the human body.

Our body is not, as I first assumed, simply an assortment of bones held together by muscles around a central pack of organs. Rather, it is a fabulously dynamic and responsive bodysuit of connective tissue that protects our organs and allows fluid movement of bones, joints, and muscles. Research suggests that our fascia, in contrast to how we once thought of it—as sheets of unfeeling tissue—can actually experience pain or pleasure and communicate sensory information directly to our brain, much like our skin, muscles, and joints do. As Dr. Langevin points out, connective tissue pathways are what connect any two points of our entire body, something you can't say about bones or muscles.

"This network is so extensive and ubiquitous," Dr. Langevin wrote in *The Scientist* in 2013, "that if we were to lose every organ, muscle, bone, nerve, and blood vessel in our bodies, we would still maintain the same shape: our 'connective tissue body.'"[35]

Increasingly clear from the research is the fact that this "connective tissue body" is what we can thank for our proper movement. We can explain the purpose of ligaments and tendons, but these discrete parts are all somewhat isolated from one another without the communication and linking action of connective tissue. We have to expand our understanding of the *entire* connective tissue network to help us learn how to keep our bodies healthy.[36]

Unhealthy fascia causes discomfort and pain in several ways. For example, with back pain, sometimes our fascia seems to be pinching, causing quite serious discomfort that cannot be easily relieved. Fascia is often described as the natural sleeve of the muscle, and just as it would be uncomfortable (or even painful) to spend the whole day with a sweater sleeve twisted around our arm, pinching fascia needs to be adjusted when we don't feel comfortable in our bodysuit. Often, fascia can be straightened out in exactly the same way we correct a twisted sweater sleeve: with a few wiggles and rotations of the arm. When getting dressed, with just a few movements we can smooth out an offending sleeve. Wiggling during warm-ups and doing a few rotations of the joint can similarly solve fascia discomfort.

People sometimes claim their fascia is "twisted" when they experience a pinching type of pain (usually in the back, hips, and thighs). What some refer to as twisted fascia is most likely *congealed* fascia (because fascia cannot twist). Layers of fascia in the painful area are adhering or "gluing" to surrounding tissue, which causes an uncomfortable tugging sensation. If not "unglued," that adhesion can lead to chronic pain. While a fascia therapist can help you differentiate fascia pain from a muscle or tendon injury (and in case of any confusion, please consult a therapist), doing ESSENTRICS can help you begin to loosen those fascial adhesions, allowing your body to release that tension and congestion.

Perhaps most promising in all the recent research on fascia is the fact that connective tissue not only gets stretched by external forces during exercise but also *responds* to that movement itself. Careful, gentle movement hydrates and heals connective tissue while working to offset inflammation. In an animal study published in 2016 in the *Journal of Cell Biology*, Dr. Langevin and her team demonstrated that stretching directly reduced the thickness of inflammatory lesions, lowered the level of neutrophils (white blood cells released during inflammation), and caused the connective tissue to release resolvin RvD1, one of the body's most potent anti-inflammatory chemicals.[37]

Gentle, full-body stretching and strengthening rejuvenates all the connective tissue simultaneously. The revelation that the techniques I have developed are ideally suited to helping increase that full-body communication, maintaining and enhancing the health of connective tissue, and reducing inflammation, has been incredibly exciting and rewarding for me. Let's talk more about how ESSENTRICS can tap into connective tissue's miraculous healing functions.

HOW MOVEMENT ORGANIZES AND REJUVENATES FASCIA

Connective tissue that surrounds and separates muscle tissue has an inherent elastic storage quality, much like the energy stored in a stretched rubber band that's about to be released. You can see how that energy potential is stored in the pattern of its collagen fibers. Healthy tissue actually has a two-dimensional weave that reminds me of the fishnet stockings I wore during the 1970s. If you looked at that weave through a microscope, you'd also see undulations called "crimp." Kids and active people of all ages have both that fishnet stocking weave and crimp in their tissues, which provide elastic storage, giving them their natural, spontaneous bounciness. Think of gazelles, kangaroos, and jackrabbits, whose long, high jumps are powered by the elastic energy stored in their extended tendons. Our tendons have a similar kinetic energy storage capacity—we use it when we jump, dance, run, and even walk. When our tendons are hydrated and pliable, we are able to naturally "spring" into action.

Over time, the tissue weave of inactive or sedentary people slowly deforms and the fibers lose their organization; they appear chaotic, lacking any sense of order, with a marked reduction in the crimp formation.[38] This combination translates into a loss of springiness and elastic recoil. You can see the difference in the diagram below.

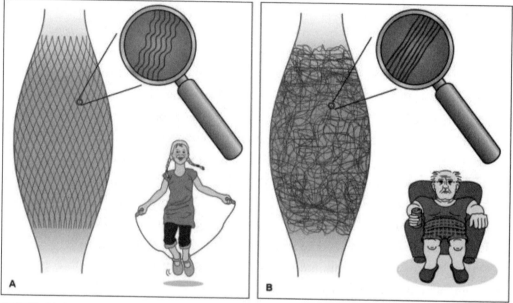

Credit: ©fascialnet.com

The wonderful news is that our natural youthful bounce, or elastic storage, can be substantially recovered through proper exercise. Research has shown that regular gentle exercise, over time, can reorganize tissue fibers and induce the return of that molecular crimp—yet one more example of how movement changes your body on the cellular level, reversing the degeneration that sometimes accompanies aging.[39]

But we have to remember that this change won't happen overnight! Muscle rejuvenation occurs much more quickly than connective tissue rejuvenation. If you've been inactive for a long time and have lost muscle mass, your muscles can be rebuilt long before your connective tissue regains its elasticity. This mismatched rate of recovery often creates frustration and can set the stage for injury.

Fascia reflects the shape of the muscle it is surrounding. If a muscle becomes compressed or shortened through overtraining, or atrophies from inactivity, the surrounding fascia will gradually shrink, too. This shrinkage is one reason why our bodies change shape over time. Fascia also reflects excess weight gain, as the superficial fascia directly under the skin and surrounding the fat cells expands with increased fat mass—but, thankfully, will usually revert to its original level of tension if the weight is lost!

As we focus on improving our fitness, we often sense our strength increase and see weight decrease much sooner than we can see any changes to our body's shape. Almost any exercise strengthens muscles relatively rapidly, because muscle activity stimulates the calorie-burning mitochondria within them, helping us to drop several pounds in a short time. Fascia renewal is a whole different story, however, taking much longer to produce visible changes. It can take months of full-body stretching and strengthening before you can see the remodeling effects of both connective tissue and muscle. However, eventually they will result in the outward appearance of the longer, leaner silhouette you can already feel inside.

As you stretch, you may think to yourself, "I feel the stretch in my muscles," but it is far more likely that you are feeling strain in your connective tissue. As mentioned before, we have about 10 times the number of sensory nerves in the fascia around the muscle than in the muscle itself. If you feel stiff after doing a stretching workout, you may mistakenly believe that stretching doesn't work for you, or that you are genetically predisposed to be stiff. Nonsense! Slow body-shape changes are simply an indication of atrophied fascia. I know that it's easy to feel discouraged, especially after many years of inactivity and atrophied fascia, if results are slow in coming. Try to stay positive, and remember: If you maintain a full-body stretching and strengthening workout, you *will* reshape your body. As a bonus for your efforts, know that improvements to fascia, which result in increased mobility and a sleeker form, are cumulative. Any gains made to the health of connective tissue will yield long-lasting results and a sleek new you.

The rehabilitation of connective tissue cannot be rushed; changing your connective tissue is a long-term project. As you get to know your body, you'll learn where your muscles and your connective tissue have become tight, and you can make conscious choices to exercise those areas extra gently.

STIFFNESS AND INFLEXIBILITY: THE IMPORTANCE OF THE OILY BATH

The stretchy connective tissue that forms a protective web surrounding every tissue in the body, all the way down to the cellular level, is only one aspect of fascia. Day and night, every cell, muscle, nerve, bone, and joint in the body is also bathed in fascia's lubricating oily bath, nourishing the surface of our muscles, cells, and joints, and preventing friction from occurring as we move. Scientists call this oily bath "the extracellular matrix," created by metabolically active stem cells called fibroblasts. These fibroblasts build and maintain the majority of the body's connective tissue, and one of their most important tasks is to excrete water and fibers (mostly collagen and some elastin) that make up the oily bath. Water is a powerful conductor, so the oily bath serves as a conduit for fascia's intercellular communication while it also lubricates the outer membranes of the cells of our muscles, preventing them from adhering to one another. Without this lubrication, our cells would stick together, making us stiff and rigid. We desperately need this lubrication so that our nerves, tendons, and ligaments can move effortlessly.

What's the first thing you say when your back feels stiff, or you can no longer touch your toes? "I'm getting so old!" Indeed, stiffness is considered one of the most common signs of aging. When people are stiff, even something as simple as stretching an arm above the head can become challenging, as does walking up stairs and bending down, among many other aspects of normal daily activity. The hardening of fascia is just one cause of stiffness, but it can be prevented, slowed down, or reversed with regular exercise. We may feel like the Tin Man in *The Wizard of Oz*—and, like the Tin Man, we need our joints to be lubricated in order to move freely. For this method of lubrication to work, we must move constantly, to help the oil maintain its liquid form and to allow for absorption. If we don't move, the oily bath that is intended as a means of lubricating our bodies can have the opposite, unintended effect.

If you use coconut oil in your kitchen, you know that when it's left sitting unused for a period of time, it will harden. This is also true of the oily bath of an inactive, sedentary person. If you are sedentary, the lubricating oils can harden, effectively securing the ligaments, nerves, or tendons inside the sheath, leaving you feeling tight, stiff—and old. If you ever use rich hand cream, you know that if you don't rub your hands together, the cream will stay on the surface of your skin and not be absorbed. The oily bath is the same: oil not constantly softened through movement and absorbed into the body will stay on the surface of the joints and muscles until it solidifies, becoming hard and thick. Like hand cream, the oily bath needs to be melted through the friction of movement in order to be rubbed in and absorbed.

When we sleep, we remain nearly immobile for up to 8 hours, but the lubrication of our cells does not stop. When we wake up, we need to move around in order to stimulate the oil that had been bathing our bodies while we slept, to actively make it absorb into our cells. The natural stretching that we instinctively do upon waking up is helpful, but it's not enough. The more out of shape a person is, the less likely he or she is to move sufficiently, and the less thoroughly the oil will be absorbed. This leads to a vicious circle: As the oil hardens, it makes the person feel stiffer and perhaps less willing or able to exercise. Many people find themselves on this slippery slope of premature aging and loss of mobility.

And it's not just age that leads to this stiffness—sometimes when we experience a minor injury or bruise, we are inclined to baby the injured area. We believe that we need to protect an injury and give it time to heal. But unless a doctor advises us otherwise, immobility is often the *worst* thing we can do! Protecting a minor injury often leads to a much graver one.

Movement is essential for healing; nonmovement puts us on a trajectory that leads to a hardening of the body's lubricating oil, cell atrophy, and stiffness in all of the surrounding areas. Immobility begins a chain reaction in which stiffness leads to more stiffness, and the end result could be a seemingly endless path of chronic pain. Clients often tell me that a current serious injury had its genesis in a smaller, treatable injury that was never encouraged to heal properly. That minor injury most likely didn't heal sufficiently because, with all good intentions, they had stopped moving after they became injured.

Unhealthy fascia is often caused by:

1. atrophy

2. immobility

3. dehydration

4. "glued" or congealed fascia (fascia layers that have adhered to themselves or other body parts)

5. injury and accidents

6. surgery and internal scarring

If you suffer a minor injury, you need to stay active; you need to continue to melt your body's hardened oil with regular and *gentle* full-body exercise. I always emphasize gentleness because rough exercise can often end up causing or aggravating injuries. Think of pulling an old bandage off a cut and ripping part of the scab with it. We don't want to tear any muscles, ligaments, fascia, or tendons. By moving gently on a daily basis, you begin to soften the hardened oil.

Mother Nature's oily bath was intended to keep the shafts of muscles, nerves, ligaments, and tendons lubricated and moving freely throughout our lives; it was never intended to solidify and restrict our movement. Let's not toss away one of Mother Nature's most generous gifts! Movement is essential to keeping all the various body parts functioning, and the oily bath is an essential part of staying pain-free, comfortably mobile, and young.

MOVEMENTS TO ENRICH YOUR CONNECTIVE TISSUE

The dynamic stretching and full-body movements of ESSENTRICS engage, stretch, and hydrate our connective tissue as very few other programs do. I know this is one reason that our participants say they have regained lost energy and suppleness along with their youthful vitality and full range of motion.

The following exercises are especially relevant to connective tissue, including the sheets of deep fascia in our torso. But almost any ESSENTRICS exercise or sequence can be adjusted to focus on connective tissue simply by doing the movements slowly and gently, while being aware that the sensation you feel while stretching should be pleasurable and never painful. The slow speed helps you to stop moving before you feel any extreme discomfort; those sensations are your body warning you to avoid potential damage. Healing should feel good! Pain is a message that something is wrong, so we want to stop before we make that "something" worse.

Connective tissue exercises should be done slowly, lovingly, continuously, and deliberately. Slow movements through a gentle range of motion increase lubrication of both the fascia and the joints. Joints will produce more fluid, and as the fascia is hydrated, tension within it will be released. If at a certain point in the movement you feel a twinge of discomfort, stop, then resume at the pace—or place—at which you feel no discomfort.

As you move, visualize your connective tissue fibers as they stretch then shrink, returning to their original shape; imagine their tight-fitting lubricated sleeves sliding over one another easily. As you move, you're rebooting the fascia encasing the muscles. The return of the spring in your step is a sign that you're starting to rebuild the crimp pattern in your connective tissue, enhancing the capacity of your tissues to store kinetic energy and to provide elasticity in your movements.

Again, please try to remember that all connective tissue reshapes slowly over time; for the better if you exercise correctly or the worse if you don't. Stiffness of your fascia reflects the years of your life during which you may have had poor habits, from overtraining to a sedentary lifestyle. If that's the case, you will need considerable time and patience to reverse the shape your tissue has taken. Every person is different; there is no hard-and-fast rule that dictates how long it will take you to change your body. What I can promise you is that as long as you keep exercising on a daily basis, you *will* experience positive results.

Ligaments: Ligaments are limited in their natural stretch to under 6 percent. The goal is not to increase their length but to maintain, or regain, their pliability. This is done by carefully moving—*not stretching*—the joints through their range of motion.

The best exercises for rejuvenating ligaments are in chapters 12, 13, 14, and 17, notably

Fingers, Wrists, and Hands (page 185)

Pliés with Heel Raisers (page 187)

Barre Footwork (page 194–95)

Chair Work for Hips (page 209)

Chair Stretch for the Psoas (page 210–11)

Calf and Soleus (page 215)

Footwork exercises (pages 257–59)

Fascia: To exercise our fascia, we need to slowly and consciously stretch and strengthen every muscle in our body. This calls for a complex variety of large and small movements involving rotating, bending, reaching, and turning in every possible direction you can. The best movements are ones that gently twist your spine in every natural direction—forward, sideways, slightly backward, and rotationally. I've made it easy for you with the exercises and sequences in this book, many of which are ideal for a deep fascia workout. Among the best are

Open Chest Swan Sequence for Posture (page 137–41)

Baby Stretch (page 135)

Pulling Weeds Sequence (page 162)

Washing Windows (page 190)

Shoulder Blast Sequence (page 223–25)

Spinal Rolls (page 242)

Single-Arm Figure 8 (page 240–41)

Pliés for Hip, Knee, and Torso Mobility (page 236)

Diagonal Windmills (page 243)

MUSCLE CHAINS COMMUNICATE THE MOVEMENT

Our skeletal muscles move the bones and joints; they are attached directly to the bones by the tendons. We have 650 skeletal muscles in our body, all differing in size and shape according to their function and duty. The brain is like the puppet master, using the muscles as strings to lift our bones like the wooden parts of a marionette.

Our muscles are made of thousands of cells bundled together, cells that need to slide around one another as we stretch or contract our muscles, each working independently and as part of a coordinated system. The bones of our arms are attached to other bones by an intricate array of muscles that run in varying patterns, from the elbows to the front and back ribs, over and under the shoulders, and into the spine. Just to attach the arms to the torso and make them work requires a phenomenal number of muscles. Even when all the muscles are working perfectly, it takes only one to give us trouble by getting injured.

We create movement with this complex series of levers and pulleys that controls our bones under the direction of signals from our brain, somewhat like a puppeteer controls the motion of a marionette. Perhaps the best way we can envision how interconnected the musculoskeletal system is to think of our very modern marionette-like technology— robotics. Scientists have recently developed state-of-the-art robotic arms and legs connected directly to the brain to replace the amputated limbs of veterans and accident victims. It has taken decades of research and millions of dollars in funding to make a robotic arm capable of such simple tasks as holding a pen, shaking someone's hand, or holding a glass of water without breaking the glass, all from the commands of the person's neurological system. The reason this technology has been so difficult to develop is that every single movement in the human body is the result of millions of messages from the brain. Even the smallest movements, like lifting your little finger or smiling, require a chain reaction of muscles acting in concert. When a muscle is injured, all the other components of that muscle chain will also be affected, and your range of movement will be hindered in ways you might not expect.

During any one day of our life, we make hundreds, even thousands of movements, each involving different sets of muscle chains. Movements as simple as standing up, sitting down, getting into and out of bed, and brushing our teeth all require the use of various sets of muscle chains. We take these simple movements for granted, but each one of them is deceptively complex, requiring that our 650 muscles—as well as our ligaments and joints—remain active and strong.

JOINTS MAKE MOVEMENT POSSIBLE

The ESSENTRICS technique is designed to engage the full body, with special attention paid to the most connective-tissue-concentrated parts of our body: our joints. The ankles, knees, and feet, and elbows, wrists, and fingers house the majority of joints in the body. Each of these is loaded with connective tissue of all types: cartilage, fascia, oily bath, tendons, and ligaments. Just think about everything your fingers enable you to do—yet there are few muscles in your fingers that do the work! Primarily just bones, fascia, oily water, tendons, and ligaments. To prevent atrophy and immobility, all this connective tissue needs to be exercised on a regular basis, especially to prevent the pain and discomfort of arthritis and osteoporosis.

While many exercise programs virtually ignore the feet, toes, hands, and fingers, ESSENTRICS focuses on them, directly and indirectly, through different sequences of movements. This focus not only helps ensure healthy joints and the pliability of the resident ligaments, but also helps prevent arthritis in the hands and feet, one of the most common conditions associated with aging.

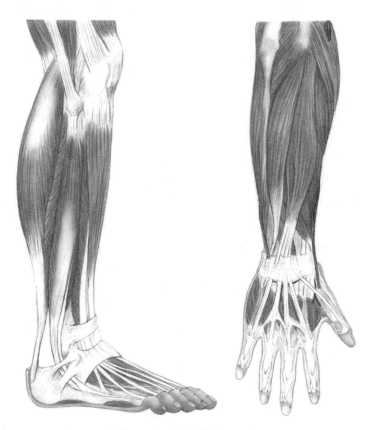

The darker color represents muscle tissue and the lighter color represents the location of tendons, cartilage, and ligaments. Notice that the knee, ankle, foot, wrist, and fingers are mainly white, because they are primarily connective tissue. Knees, hands, and feet are where most arthritis and joint pain is experienced, making these connective tissue conditions.

Credits: © Asklepios Medical Atlas / Science Source (*left*) © Stocktrek Images / Science Source (*right*)

Joints are found at the meeting of two bones, attached by ligaments and moved by our musculature. Joints come in many different shapes and sizes, from finger joints—which are small and relatively straightforward—to wrist, hip, knee, ankle, and shoulder joints—which are large and complex. Each joint plays a vital role in the mobility of our individual parts, and each is necessary to the mobility of the body as a whole. The muscle activates the function of the joint—so when muscles are tight or imbalanced, that directly affects the joint's range of motion. All range of motion is controlled or animated by the muscle functions of the joint and pliability of the ligaments.

Where two bones meet, we have various types of spongy cushion, like buffers, cartilage, and disks, all of which are necessary to prevent the surface of the two bones from grinding against each other like sandpaper. If the muscles and ligaments atrophy, the joints become compressed and the cartilage or disks damaged. Protecting this buffer is essential to lasting joint health.

If your finger joints feel stiff or painful, you'll struggle to hold a knife and fork, get dressed, button buttons, or tie your shoelaces. If your hip joints are stiff, you'll struggle to sit down and stand up. These are signs that the cartilage between your joints is wearing away, and the joints are increasingly reduced to raw bone on bone. Even the simple task of walking will be painful and strained. We need our joints to have full range of motion in order to be pain-free, to function on a basic level, or even just to feel comfortable in our bodies.

Joints also require lubrication, in the same way a piston or door hinge does, which is provided by the synovial fluid found in sacs that surround every joint. This lubrication allows our joints to slide smoothly and effortlessly in specific directions. When they're strong and flexible, our joints are largely self-sufficient entities, requiring minimal upkeep to function properly for decades. They are designed to remain healthy for the duration of our lives. Unless they are damaged from neglect, trauma, or disease, they will not disintegrate on their own.

Joints consist of strong durable material that is, in theory, able to last a lifetime, which insinuates that "age-related" joint damage is a misnomer. So why are joint pain and damage so remarkably common? Let's dig a little deeper.

LIGAMENT PLIABILITY IS THE ANSWER

The ability of connective tissue to store energy is what helped humans evolve to the point where we can throw 100 mph fastballs. In a 2013 letter published in the journal

Nature, researchers from Harvard described how humans evolved their blazingly fast throwing capacity thanks in large part to the energy storage potential of their shoulder tendons and ligaments. The researchers explained that when a pitcher bends his arm to cock the ball back, certain tendons and ligaments are stretched and store the energy (like an elongated rubber band). Then, when the pitcher releases the ball, the energy is released along with it, and the ball shoots out as if launched by a slingshot.[40]

Now, granted, these are professional athletes using their ligaments in an extreme way that nature probably did not intend! But this does show the tremendous potential of our connective tissue to do amazing things with that stored energy.

Normally, ligaments are tight, stiff bands of a collagen-rich connective tissue. The primary purpose of ligaments is to attach one bone to another while they support our joints, keeping them safely aligned to prevent the joints from wobbling unstably. Without the support of our ligaments, our hips would sway uncontrollably with every movement, our knees would buckle inward or outward with every step, and our ankles would collapse as our feet touched the ground. So ligaments must be sufficiently tight to resist the pressure of the full body's weight without stretching beyond their natural limited degree of elasticity.

A ligament at its healthiest should be pliable enough to allow its supporting joint a range of motion from 4 to 6 degrees. However, if the ligaments are *never* moved, as in someone with a sedentary lifestyle, they gradually harden and dry out, losing their 4 to 6 degrees of flexibility. This is visible when people who had previously been mobile and active, but have now become more sedentary, can no longer bend their knees, open their legs sideways, or flex their ankles.

Dried, stiff, atrophied ligaments are a clear sign of premature aging. To reverse this, the ligaments must be exercised extremely carefully to prevent tearing or stretching beyond their 6 degrees of pliability. To regain ligament pliability, we have to work diligently and carefully. We are never trying to increase their flexibility; we do not want ligaments to be flexible, we want them to be *pliable*. Pliability means that they are capable of moving, whereas flexibility insinuates that there is a lengthening and a recoiling action (as in muscles). Stretched ligaments will make our joints unstable and injury-prone. Pliable ligaments give us mobility and support.

When ligaments get stiff, they restrict the movement of the surrounding tissue—in much the same way a cast or brace does—leading, inevitably, to muscle weakness and atrophy; we can barely move the affected joints. Consider the strongest joint in the body, the ankle. Think about the job it has to do, supporting the full weight of your body all day long. We need strength and mobility in our ankles so that they can safely bear the burden of our weight as we walk, run, jump, or just carry on our daily lives. But when ankles stiffen from tight ligaments, walking becomes difficult, as we need mobility in the ankle joints to help in the propulsion of our bodies. The stiffness that started in our ankles causes a negative chain reaction up the legs and into the knees, hips, and spine, causing muscular imbalances, poor posture, and chronic aches and pains. Indeed, one of the major chains in our body begins with our toes and goes all the way up to our neck muscles. Any tension or immobility in the toes hinders ankle mobility, leading to stiffened calf muscles, and quickly spreads to the rest of the chain, causing stiffness and pain as far up as the back and neck.

Try the following experiment: Tighten your ankle joints so that they cannot move. Then try walking with no movement in the ankles. The first thing you will notice is that you cannot walk very fast. You will find yourself shuffling like an old person. You should also notice that after about 10 or 15 steps, your knees, hips, and back start hurting.

Try the same experiment with your fingers: Lock your fingers and then try to close a button, write a note, or pick up a cup! Losing mobility is very scary, isn't it?

Even in the fitness industry, the importance of maintaining pliable (not flexible) ligaments, particularly in the feet, has long been overlooked. Tightness is assumed to be caused by muscular inflexibility, but in reality inflexible ligaments are what lead to inflexible muscles. Tight ligaments slow us down and bring about arthritis and the possible need for joint replacement.

The good news is that it is preventable (and, depending on the degree, reversible) through gentle movement. The solution is always the same: Gently increase the movement of the toe and ankle ligaments, and a positive chain reaction will ripple through the adjoining muscles, loosening them and relieving stiffness and pain.

JOINTS CAN BE PAINFUL . . . AND EXPENSIVE!

Nothing says old age like creaky joints. When we hear this telltale creak, it's often accompanied by deterioration in the joints and the beginning of chronic pain, which can become debilitating. When joints are functioning well, all our movements are fluid and efficient, and we don't even notice which joints are involved in which movements. But when joints are diseased or damaged, every movement becomes torturous. Paraphrasing Joni Mitchell, we don't know what we've got till it's gone—we never really appreciate our joints and all that they do for us until they are no longer functioning properly!

When people suffer from joint problems, they naturally look for the fastest, easiest ways to relieve their pain. However, if the root cause is not resolved, the damage will get progressively worse. And the root cause is not aging but a lifetime of bad habits, including

Being sedentary. Couch potatoes are actually at a greater risk of suffering from joint problems than are weekend warriors or hard-driving athletes. The main reason sedentary people experience more joint pain and arthritis is atrophy: wasting of muscle tissue caused by disuse. With atrophy, muscles lose their elasticity, becoming smaller, drier, and stiffer; their shrinkage causes the joints to compress, eliminating the space necessary for synovial fluid to lubricate the joints. The result is a disintegration of the disk or cartilage, leading to a grating of bone on bone that is both painful and debilitating—a condition known as arthritis. Arthritis makes any activity, even something as benign as walking across a room, excruciatingly painful (often leading to hip and knee joint replacement as well as spinal fusions).

For sedentary folks, movement is an amazingly simple and powerful solution to an otherwise complicated problem. If you've been sedentary for a while, do not be discouraged by your perceived limitations—just begin today, right where you are, at home. Get up and walk around, making sure you gently bend and straighten all your joints. Wiggle your toes and fingers, rotate your ankles and shoulders, bend your knees and elbows. And then build on that with some gentle ESSENTRICS exercises, and you will feel considerable improvement quite rapidly. (See "Are You Sedentary?" on page 36.)

Being overweight. Often, excess body weight goes hand in hand with a sedentary lifestyle, one causing or exacerbating the other. While excess weight may seem like an easy scapegoat for joint problems, people who have lost weight will tell you how much better their joints feel after they've shed some extra pounds. The compression caused by excess weight eventually flattens the joints' natural cushions, squeezing out the lubricating synovial fluid sacs and leading to the grinding of bone on bone that we so desperately want to avoid. Losing weight alleviates the compression of the joints, restoring a space for the fluid sacs to spread lubrication.

Often, obese or overweight people ask me what exercises they can do to relieve their hip and knee pain. I gently suggest that if they lose the weight, the pain will go away. It's true—I promise!

Poor running or walking habits. A sedentary lifestyle is much more dangerous to joints than any sport or activity could ever be. That said, poor running and walking habits are another major cause of joint damage. If a runner runs heavily on a hard surface, such as concrete, they will eventually develop joint trauma. Runners and walkers tend to respond to joint pain by purchasing state-of-the-art running shoes, in the vain hope that these will provide the amount of cushioning required to soften the impact, thus sparing their joints. But even the best running shoe is incapable of cushioning against that slamming effect.

In addition to impact trauma with a heavy walking or running stride, there is also the problem of muscles constantly contracting and never lengthening. No shoe, no matter how ingenious the design, can protect against the repetitive shortening of the muscles that occurs with a runner's stride. The initial cause of the pain, before the actual joint head gets damaged, is shortened muscles. Shortened muscles cause the bones to squeeze the joints tightly together. The combination of damage from repetitive impact to the head of the joint and the shortened muscles squeezing the joints together leaves no space for the synovial fluid to lubricate the joint, as well as no room for the cartilage to slide smoothly—and this condition is the precursor to arthritis.

With conditions like joint damage that becomes arthritis, we generally resort to treating our *symptoms* rather than addressing the underlying *causes*. Perhaps this is due to our defeatist mentality about aging: We assume pain is part of the process. We opt for a fast and simple "solution," reaching for an anti-inflammatory or painkiller to mask the problem, and, like magic, the pain is gone. Ah, but the trouble that caused the pain and the continued damage isn't gone. Unless we treat the cause, the pain (and possibly those pills) will be with us for the rest of our lives.

Our joints are truly designed to last a lifetime. But even though the repercussions from poor habits and wear and tear are not apparent until we are older, the damage starts accumulating when we are young. Years of poor walking and running habits will eventually wear down a joint to the point that replacement surgery is required. Prevention is the best solution. Knowing how to be light on your feet is the first step toward preventing joint damage, and it takes only 10 minutes to learn how to walk lightly. Parents should teach their children as well, just as we teach them the daily habit of brushing and flossing their teeth. (Look on YouTube for instructional videos by physical therapists or exercise physiologists.) Runners should also learn good running technique. Pulling out of the joint with strengthened full-body muscles is the only permanent way to protect joints from impact damage. If you get rid of the impact, you get rid of the root cause of the damage.

Sports injuries. A great deal of joint damage that I've seen in professional sports is reversible, and nearly all of it is preventable. Athletes in many sports, including soccer, hockey, tennis, football, and basketball, tend to develop very tight muscles, which cause undue compression of the joints (particularly in the hip, knee, shoulder, and spine). Over time, the compression takes a serious toll on the cartilage, causing damage.

The training of young athletes too often focuses solely on the development of strength and neglects the need for range of motion. After decades of working with high-performance athletes, I can tell you that many athletes receive almost no dynamic flexibility or muscle decompression training. As a result, their joints grind together with every movement, and their muscles and tendons are prone to tears and strains.

Range of motion of any joint is vital to athletic performance and the prevention of injuries. Some coaches try to prevent injuries with yoga or static stretches, but that type of stretching isn't effective for this purpose. Yoga holds static poses, and static stretching actually creates unbalanced muscle development and shortened instead of lengthened muscles. Eccentric exercise strengthens the muscles while simultaneously stretching and lengthening them. Dynamic range of motion stretching can not only prevent injury and enhance performance; it can save careers and create champions! After a few weeks of dynamic flexibility or eccentric stretching, I have seen many of these young athletes go on to win world championships and Olympic medals.

Interestingly, the reason athletes damage their joints is identical to the reason normal people do. The only difference is that the damage in athletes presents itself much earlier. Most amateur athletes and weekend warriors jump straight into physical activity with little to no preparation. With cold and tight muscles, they lace up their skates or put on their shoes and, within minutes, transition from a near-static state to one of intense activity. This is a recipe for disaster, and as they age they find themselves saddled with debilitating joint pain.

I've found it challenging to persuade athletes to delay starting right away, especially when they are young, but the small amount of time spent doing a dynamic warm-up routine could spare them weeks, months, or even years of pain and inactivity resulting from damaged joints. Prevention needs to be encouraged, embraced, and emphasized, at all levels and ages.

HOW ESSENTRICS PROTECTS JOINTS AND HEALS CONNECTIVE TISSUE

The dynamic eccentric stretching in ESSENTRICS pulls apart the joints while strengthening them, thus preventing joint damage in the first place. Pulling apart the joints creates a space for the lubricating and healing synovial fluid to enter. This fluid prevents grinding on the joint while also healing any damage. Eccentric stretching also prevents the squeezing effect that is the actual cause of the pain and damage.

You may need to take some time to relieve compressed joints and rebuild atrophied tissue, but the reward is worth the effort. Have faith in your body's proven ability to heal itself. Be realistic in your expectations—slowing down the aging process is, in many ways, as good as reversing it!

And remember: When we stretch, we're stretching not only muscle but also our dynamic and responsive connective tissue. Long-term and regular stretching has an amazing impact on the architecture of the fascia, helping reduce inflammation and maintain your connective tissue's youthful elasticity. Just as squeezing a damp sponge moves the moisture from one place to another, the act of stretching pushes fascial liquid from areas where it may have congealed, dispersing the fluids, keeping the tissue moist and pliable, and refreshing other neglected areas of our connective tissue that don't have adequate hydration.

Now let's turn our attention to flexibility—what it is, why it's important, and how the ESSENTRICS program can help us relax into new levels of strength and flexibility.

PART II

HOW WE STAY YOUNG AND HEALTHY

CHAPTER 5

STRETCH IT OUT

FLEXIBILITY IS THE
FOUNTAIN OF YOUTH

In the standard approach to stiffness and joint pain, we tend to treat the symptoms and not the underlying causes. This shortsighted approach always makes me think of an old dancer's saying: "You are only as loose as your tightest muscle." We need to make sure that every muscle is equally stretched and strengthened in relationship to the surrounding muscles, not only to manage pain and stiffness but also to perform at our peak abilities.

A few years ago I worked with prima ballerina Anik Bissonnette. Anik had been in Moscow performing *Giselle* as a guest artist of the Bolshoi Ballet, one of the world's premiere ballet companies. She had suffered for years from chronic hip pain and to control the pain, she was under the permanent care of a company physiotherapist and osteopath.

During a break in the middle of her ballet tour, Anik joined my team in Mexico for a two-week film shoot for the latest Classical Stretch DVD. During that time, she didn't do any ballet classes and did only Classical Stretch. She was worried that Classical Stretch wasn't challenging enough to keep her at the high level of physical fitness she required as a ballerina. While she felt much better, she thought that she would surely be out of shape when she returned to the company after her two weeks with us.

Much to her surprise, two things happened by the end of the two-week filming: Her chronic hip pain disappeared (never to return!) and when she got back to the company, she was stronger than when she had left.

During those two weeks, we were not doing any special exercises for Anik's hips; she was simply doing regular Classical Stretch workouts that are designed to rebalance the full body, the same DVD workouts that are marketed and sold to everyday exercisers. We didn't work on the symptoms, but rather, in following the ESSENTRICS program so diligently for two weeks, we were able to completely resolve the underlying cause of the problem. This turnaround is a perfect example of how rebalancing exercises can work their magic through all the muscle chains of the body.

HOW MUSCLE CHAINS GET SEVERED

I often share this image with my trainees: When a door is loose on its hinge, it hangs off center, swinging awkwardly and closing imperfectly. The hinge could be loose because of something as simple as a screw not being tight enough, and that small problem can lead to a major problem. If the screw doesn't get tightened, the door eventually becomes so unbalanced that it will be difficult to close and could end up ruining its frame or structure. What grew into a serious structural problem could have been easily prevented and corrected by tightening the loose screw in the first place.

As with the broken door and the loose screw, if any of the muscles of a joint are too tight or too weak to hold the joint comfortably in correct alignment, the tightest muscle will pull the joint out of alignment, unbalancing it and ultimately causing pain and injury. I've found that balancing the entire muscular structure simultaneously is one of the most miraculous-feeling and rewarding elements of these workouts—and one that has the biggest impact on people's quality of life.

TRACING THE PATH OF MUSCLE CHAINS

Each muscle and each bone has a role to play in shaping your body and facilitating movement. Just to be able to hold your head on top of your shoulders without letting it fall over requires the support of dozens of muscles, soft tissue, and the bones of the cervical spine. Think about it: How amazing is it that you can hold up the heavy weight of your head, all day, without compressing your spine? Even with this constant pressure on our spines, only a few people suffer from back pain. We owe a huge debt of gratitude to the strength of our muscles.

The brilliant design of your body becomes even more impressive when you stop to think about how many moving parts make up a human being and how complex a pulley and lever system is needed to make any movement smooth and easy. We've talked about how muscle chains work, and how each muscle in the chain affects others. But technically, muscle chains are only indirectly attached, because muscles attach to bones. Each bone in our body has a muscle pulling at the front and back end. In fact, with 620 muscles and only 200 bones, often several muscles are attached to the same bone, each pulling in a slightly different direction.

Small muscle chains move our fingers, turn our heads, and bend our knees. Large chains go from our toes to our fingertips. When it comes to maintaining a youthful feeling in our body and remaining free of pain, all chains—large and small—are equally important.

In what I call a balanced body, all of the 620 muscles are equally strong and flexible. But muscle chains can be broken or interrupted in several ways. When a chain is broken, only the sides that the muscles are pulling are activated; the muscles on the other side cannot move. The consequences of broken muscle chains can be very severe, leading to stiffness and eventually atrophy on the side that is not being pulled.

Common causes of an interruption of the flow of signals in a muscle chain include

- scar tissue from surgery

- large bruises

- broken bones

- torn or injured muscles, ligaments, or tendons

- sprains and strains

- back pain

- sciatica

- shin splints

Sometimes the flow of information is completely severed, as in a spinal cord injury or a cut tendon, and sometimes it is partially interrupted. Sometimes overbuilding certain muscle groups can create imbalances in which certain muscles overpower others, resulting in atrophy of the weaker muscles.

Lower body blockages. I see this a great deal with professional hockey players and Olympic skiers, whose hamstrings, glutes, and quads are so tight that their calf muscles can't move. This condition leads to groin injuries, as the chains connecting the groin muscles are unable to move efficiently. The rigid hamstrings block the chain that flows into the groin muscles, resulting in extremely tight, often pulled groin muscles.

The feet and ankles are the starting point of a major chain that goes from toes to fingers. When the ankle joints are tight or weak, there is little to no mobility in the ankles. This affects the mechanics of how we walk and how much energy we have available. Stiffness in the ankles causes tension in the calf muscles. That tension causes tension in the quadriceps, which then causes compression of the knee joints and leads to pain. Any weakness or lack of mobility will spread far and wide, causing problems in parts of the body that are seemingly unrelated to the original source of the weakness. Foot weakness can cause back pain—such is the nature of muscle chains.

Upper body blockages. Blockages of upper body muscle chains are particularly common in athletes who focus excessively on the trapezius and deltoid muscles, which in turn force the shoulders into a rounded position. The disproportionately stronger back muscles overpower the muscles of the chest, creating an imbalance in the chain that leads to poor posture and injury.

Mid-body blockages. When hip or back muscles are tight, they will often block the chains of muscles that are either above or below them. If we do not do large, full-body movements to keep these large chains strong and flexible, the result will be problems like back pain, poor posture, drooping shoulders, tight legs, and difficulty sitting down in or standing up from a chair.

When the large chains have been broken, either by lack of flexibility or by an injury, they always cause imbalances that lead to pain. These imbalances are manifested as poor posture, back pain, arthritis, and injuries. Full-body rebalancing workouts that include equal amounts of strengthening and flexibility movement are important to keep us pain-free, fully mobile, and feeling young.

Now that we have a sense of what's at stake, let's look at how we can increase our flexibility.

HOW ESSENTRICS INCREASES FLEXIBILITY

We can think of the whole body as a collection of functional groups of muscles, with those in each group having equal but opposing actions. Our muscles are arranged in specific groups, and within each group, in opposing pairs. When one muscle contracts and shortens, the opposing muscle relaxes and lengthens. For example, one group of muscles lifts your leg while the opposite group of muscles releases the leg to be lifted. Together, their actions work in harmony and, ideally, the degree of contraction in the working muscle *should be* equal to the degree of elongation in the opposing muscle. In ESSENTRICS, our muscles constantly alternate between contraction and elongation, so the muscle groups being used become equally stretched and strengthened.

Stretching, by definition, is about increasing the distance between two joints by gently pulling them apart using their adjoining muscles. Static stretches do this by isolating and stretching one set of muscles, such as the hamstrings, and do not include the surrounding muscles, such as those that run alongside the upper thigh to join at the hip. But in real life, if you move your leg, you use every one of those muscles. If those other muscles are not stretched adequately, you could stretch the hamstring all day and it wouldn't make you feel any more flexible. Your range of motion will always be determined by your least flexible muscle.

That's why, in ESSENTRICS, we use eccentric force on *all* of the muscles that surround the joint to help pull it apart. Those muscles could be long, short, flat, wide, irregular, or even triangular. But in order to make the stretch effective, they all have to be involved in the stretch.

The arrangement of the muscles around the joint dictates the direction in which we pull. For example, the knee, which is a hinge joint, swings forward and backward. The muscles on both sides of the knee hinge—the hamstrings and the quadriceps—create both forward and backward phases of the swinging motion, and both need to be equally strong and flexible so the knee can remain balanced. This ESSENTRICS approach to full-body balance has several additional benefits:

Helps broaden range of motion within each joint. While we stretch, we also rotate the joint in the middle of the stretch. By doing this rotation movement while we stretch, we activate any surrounding muscles that tend to get ignored in standard static stretching. This activation balances the joint and helps relieve pain.

Helps strengthen functional exercise skills. Throughout the exercises, we try to mirror the constant body movements that we use in real life, whether we're reaching for things on a high shelf, twisting to wave to a friend behind us, or bending down to pick up a child or a heavy bag of groceries. We do this not merely to help you do your chores more effectively; we also know that these types of everyday activities engage muscles that isolated stretches tend to miss.

Helps strengthen the mind-body connection. The exercises in ESSENTRICS are designed to follow the natural chains of the muscles in continuous circular and rotational movements. Following the natural chains of the muscles feels easy and soothing, in sync with the body's instinctive flow. The organic nature of these movements leaves you with a sense of well-being. The movements seem to be in harmony with what your body instinctively wants to do and how it wants to move. At the end of an ESSENTRICS workout, you will be likely to feel relaxed and contented, even though you've just finished a rigorous activity.

Helps strengthen the weakest links in our body. Of course, the fitness gained from following the muscle chains is as valuable as the emotional benefit. If one muscle along the chain is weaker, tighter, or in any way off balance relative to the others, all of the muscles along the chain will be affected. That's why a foot injury can cause hip problems, or an arm injury can cause shoulder problems. In order to operate at our peak, we must rebalance the entire body.

HOW TO ASSESS YOUR OWN FLEXIBILITY

When starting ESSENTRICS, most people want to know how flexible they can become. No matter what, *everybody* has the ability to gain some degree of flexibility. That said, no two people are alike—if you've never in your life been able to touch your toes, you're not likely to suddenly be able to fold yourself into a pretzel. Working from an original starting point, the average person can gain between 60 and 75 percent additional flexibility and contract the muscles an additional 25 percent by following a program like ESSENTRICS.

What we call a "muscle" is really two things:

1. The actual skeletal muscle organ, which is made up of millions of filaments of protein strands bundled together (which turn the mitochondria fuel ATP into energy)

2. Tendons that are made of fibrous connective tissue, which attaches the muscles to the bones.

You can't judge your muscles' potential flexibility on the basis of a standard flexibility test—everyone has a different potential. The differences between you and other people will be mainly due to the ratio of your skeletal muscle to tendon.

Tendons are very stiff while muscles are very supple. The skeletal muscle has the ability to contract roughly 25 percent, as it is strengthened, and extend roughly 60 to 75 percent, as it is elongated or stretched. Tendons, by contrast, are made of fibrous connective tissue and have a limited flexibility range (between 4 and 6 percent, as we discussed in Chapter 4).

We train all our instructors to assess a person's potential flexibility by using a measure we call "best resting." Best resting is the neutral point just at the start of movement. Once you begin to move, your muscles will start to contract or lengthen, indicating your neutral or resting level of flexibility prior to any significant exercise.

In judging potential flexibility, one thing we think about is the ratio of tendon length to muscle length. Some people have a lower tendon-to-muscle ratio than others. The longer your muscle is in relation to the length of your tendons, the greater your degree of potential flexibility. If you have very limited range of motion, you can assume that your tendons are longer and your muscles are shorter. If this sounds like you, you may never achieve great flexibility, but you can still improve your flexibility dramatically. And if you show a significant range of motion at your best resting position, then you can assume that your tendon-to-muscle ratio is low and that you will see very impressive changes in your flexibility by following the ESSENTRICS exercises.

Best resting depends on several factors, including your

- genetic profile

- age

- level of fitness

- ratio of tendon length to muscle length

- type of previous training

Sadly, no amount of flexibility training can change the reality of a high tendon-to-muscle ratio. You may not be able to become a gymnast or a ballerina, but you absolutely can achieve your own maximum flexibility. Everyone experiences an increased range of motion—from significant to downright astonishing—after doing these exercises for a couple of months.

Sometimes our stiffness, pain, or lack of flexibility is due not to our muscles or tendons, but to our fascia. Luckily, ESSENTRICS can help there, too.

USING ESSENTRICS TO READJUST FASCIA

We talked about fascia, one part of what I call the "oily bath," in Chapter 4. One of the most exciting side benefits of this exercise program is how well it can help to readjust fascia that is out of place.

We have two kinds of fascia, superficial and deep, which can vary in thickness and size. Sometimes fascia is described as a type of cellophane sleeve that's made up of flexible collagen tissue and fat. Fascia surrounds individual muscle fibers as well as whole muscle groups, such as the back of the neck into the shoulders, or the quadriceps into the lower back, that hold and support everything in its place. One of the largest fascia coverings in the body is described as "trousers" that cross over the knee and finish above the hips. These fascia "trousers" are thicker around the knee, thin out as they continue up the leg and hips, and then thicken again near the pelvis.

Picture what happens when you put on a sweater and the sleeve is twisted around your arm—uncomfortable, right? You wriggle and twist the cloth around your arm, and you typically can't focus on anything else until the sweater is positioned correctly. Well, fascia is often called the "sleeve" of the muscle, and it can also become twisted, pinching the muscles and causing inflammation and pain.

We often can't tell the difference between fascia pain and muscle injury, as in the case of chronic back pain or knee pain. Fascia is also the entry point of many nerves, and this factor heightens the potential for pain. Typical pain relief measures, such as heat, cold, and even painkillers, won't work—only straightening the fascia will stop the pinching and relieve the pain.

ESSENTRICS' techniques use movement within a stretch and rotation of a joint to help straighten out the twisted fascia. Sometimes all it takes is a few simple rotations of the joint to reposition the fascia correctly. When the fascia is straightened out, the pinching stops and the pain disappears.

One exception occurs when the fascia has become traumatized by injury, and develops scarring. But scarring isn't confined to acute injuries. We all develop multiple small and large scars and adhesions throughout our body, accumulating them as we go through life. Their buildup can contribute to our sense of feeling older. Luckily, gentle exercise can help us there, too.

HEALING SCAR TISSUE

When we think of scar tissue, we think of scars on the surface of our skin that we see with our naked eye, not internal scars. But most of us have more internal than external scars, as a result of the bumps, bruises, or surgeries that we experienced over many years of life. The accumulation of these scars is part of what determines our pace of aging, as it can lead to restricted movement, muscle imbalance (when we "baby" an injury), and general stiffness and chronic pain of all kinds.

Scars are the seams created to bind together two cut parts of soft tissue in order to stop bleeding. Whether the bleeding is on the surface of our skin or internal, any bleeding has to be cauterized to stop the flow of blood; the resulting seam is called a scar. What we in the antiaging business need to recognize is that scar tissue is a type of atrophied cell.

Everyone is familiar with what a cut looks like; we've all seen red blood flow out of a wound, usually followed by a clear whitish fluid. This white fluid is actually a part of our immune system that is sent to wounded areas; within minutes, the fluid crystallizes, forming a scab, which stops the bleeding. The scab looks like an ugly, brownish mound and eventually falls off, leaving behind a thin pale scar.

In order to understand how a scar interferes with the mobility of the body, we need to understand how the fibers of the body work. The fibers of body tissue run in the same direction as one another, like the threads in a piece of cloth. If you pulled a piece of cloth, it would unravel along the lines of the threads. Imagine that you sewed a thick, heavy seam (the scar) across the lines of the fabric, and then pulled on a thread: Only those threads on the side of the seam that you were pulling on would move. The threads on the other side of the seam would be blocked and immobilized by the seam.

Your body tissue works in much the same way. When you have a scar, it interferes with the movement of the muscle or skin tissue. When you pull one side, as when you lift your arm above your head, the other side won't move—a scar blocks the connection between the two sides, even interrupting major muscle chains throughout the body. The degree of interference corresponds to the size of the scar.

Soft body tissue, like skin and muscles, is made of cells that form hundreds of tissue-paper-thin layers lying on top of one another, giving the appearance of one solid, thick layer. In operations, when surgeons cut through the skin, they are in fact cutting through hundreds of individual layers of cells. Each layer is kept separate from the layer above by a lubricating fluid that prevents layers from being glued together.

The human body is very efficient in dealing with damage; it has the world's best triage unit. When we are cut, white blood cells rush to the rescue with one objective in mind: Stop the bleeding! And it's a good thing, since any cut or wound gives outside germs and bacteria easy access to the vital organs of the body through the bloodstream.

In order to seal a wound as rapidly as possible, the immune system goes into intense action, slapping on the white blood corpuscles in an attempt to stop the bleeding. The body does not try to make a perfect job of it—the only objective is to stop the bleeding. Anytime the skin is broken, whether by accident or surgery, scar tissue forms to seal the cut and bind together the spliced layers of skin or muscle. In the process, as a side effect, thousands of skin layers become glued together. The result of binding layers together is to give the skin a puckered appearance. This also leads to restricted movement between the two sides of the scar. Physical therapy is recommended to prevent the skin layers from remaining glued together, and it has to be done in the weeks immediately following surgery. But many people don't realize the importance of this part of healing and some ignore their doctors' orders. (I should know, as I am guilty of ignoring my own doctor's advice, and now I have an immobile scar on my wrist!) This is why scar tissue leaves us with less range of motion and less mobility both on the surface and internally.

Interior ripping and tearing happen from time to time during life. A bruise is a sign of internal bleeding. The process of healing a bruise is identical to that of healing a surface cut: White blood cells rush to the rescue, binding the wound and leaving behind a stiffened, albeit healed, wound. The bruise is created from the blood that escaped before the wound was sealed.

We all suffer hundreds of micro tears, cuts, and bruises over the years of our lives; we bump into a desk, trip on an uneseen object, slice our finger while cooking, take a bad fall while playing a sport. Minor accidents are unavoidable, but with each bump and bruise we develop a new scar. We accumulate quite a few scars over the course of our lives, and if we don't get rid of excess scar tissue we will become extremely stiff. Exercise helps make that scar tissue flexible again.

Some of the best exercises to get rid of scar tissue are slow, sensuous movements that mimic the body, such as cat arches or ceiling reaches. These movements are deceptively simple—we don't need a personal trainer to show us how to do them, but we do need to take the time to stretch slowly and regularly to get the maximum benefit.

Another way to help heal scar tissue is to massage the affected area in order to dislodge the layers of skin that have become glued together. The sooner we massage a scar, the less likely it is that the layers of skin will glue together. This is why doctors recommend gentle massage after surgery or trauma.

When it comes to internal scarring, a massage by a therapist can dig only so deep into our muscles. But we can replace the massaging action with gentle, rotational, twisting and turning movements. Rotational movements help to loosen internal scar tissue, sloughing off the excess debris and liberating the bound-up muscle.

A note of warning for those who don't exercise after undergoing a major surgery: I've had clients who have come to me many years after having had surgery (abdominal, knee, ankle, or spinal) and who didn't exercise or do the physical therapy their doctors prescribed. Predictably, a few years later, the entire body began to feel some degree of pain caused by the restricted movement from internal scarring. They come to me because they are suffering.

Atrophy happens to people of all ages, whether they're 15 years old or 80 years old. And while old scars and years of immobility are more difficult to treat than new wounds, we can still help to repair old injuries. In 2012, Dr. Langevin released preliminary research for three studies funded by the National Institutes of Health (NIH). These breakthroughs have opened a conversation about using dynamic stretching to prevent and heal injuries and pain.

Dr. Langevin's work showed that dynamic stretching employing a full range of motion can have an effect in regulating the tension level of connective tissue; this regulation in turn helps to relieve conditions like back pain.[41] Dynamic range of motion stretching is the same type of movement that is used in Classical Stretch, ESSENTRICS, and tai chi. This research could explain why so many people who do ESSENTRICS report reduced or totally relieved pain, and it is groundbreaking for sufferers from back pain, athletes, and physical therapists alike.

Anytime there is interference with the ability to move, there is a risk of atrophy. This

BREAST CANCER AND SCAR TISSUE

When I was 50, I had breast cancer. After my breast cancer surgery, my biggest problem was the scar tissue that had accumulated under my arm where the surgeon had removed lymph nodes. I had difficulty raising my arm even to shoulder height because doing so tugged on the scar in my underarm. I was afraid that if I pulled too hard I might reopen the incision, so I stopped raising my arm whenever I felt a tug on the scar tissue. Soon, even raising my arm to shoulder height was painful.

Fortunately, with the advice and encouragement of the physiotherapists and nurses at the Royal Victoria Hospital, I was able to work within my limits and through the pain. They showed me that I wouldn't rip the scar tissue or cause additional damage to the wound if I was careful (one of my biggest worries). I followed their advice, working within their prescribed limits, until I regained the full range of motion in my arm in about 8 weeks—but the sensations of tugging and stiffness took more than 10 years to go away. And every time I lift my arm above my head (which is every day, as it is a basic movement in my fitness program), I still feel a slight pain, though it disappears rapidly.

I realized that if an exercise specialist like me had difficulty understanding the simple instructions that breast cancer patients are given after surgery, there must be millions of women experiencing similar confusion. With support from the Royal Victoria Hospital and Novartis, I created a complete breast cancer rehabilitation workout that's available free of charge on my website (www.classicalstretch.com) for any woman who has undergone breast cancer surgery.

Once I understood the full nature of my problems, I was inspired with the confidence to push through painful rehabilitation exercises. To this day, 14 years later, every time I raise my arm above my head, I still feel a slight tug against the scar. But within seconds as I continue the stretch, the tugging sensation disappears. The scar may never go away, but I'm grateful I made sure to retain my mobility and the full use of my arms!

means that scar tissue can lead to atrophy unless we consciously move all of the tissue (both skin and muscle) surrounding the scar. Regular exercises can get rid of scar tissue and, thankfully, the movements required to release scar tissue are the easiest exercises to perform.

We've talked a lot about helping to relieve pain and increase our flexibility with the stretching component of ESSENTRICS. But the other half of the eccentric approach—to *strengthen* as we stretch—is equally important. Let's look at how we can increase our strength while simultaneously increasing the number and power of our cells' antiaging mitochondria.

CHAPTER 6

MAXIMIZE MUSCLE POWER

BOOSTING STRENGTH AND ENDURANCE

Our muscles have many jobs to perform to keep us healthy and vibrant. They move us around, give us our shape, regulate our weight, and supply us with energy. The muscular system is also designed to work in harmony with the other major systems of the body to keep them functioning efficiently. But the muscular system needs to be cared for before it can start doing its own jobs and assisting all our other systems.

Perhaps the most obvious role muscles play in our lives is the image we see every day in the mirror. Muscle and bone create the structure of our bodies. But we cannot change the shape of our bones; we have no control over the basic form that we have been born with. Neither do we have control over our height. Those qualities are determined by our genetic profile and we cannot alter them. In contrast, we can do a great deal with our muscles. We can make them strong, flexible, and lean, or rigid and bulky. Or we can ignore them entirely and just let them become weak and flabby—the choice is ours.

One thing is clear: The best way to care for our muscles is not to spend hours in the gym. Instead, the best way to strengthen, lengthen, and protect the health of our muscles is to try to simulate the way we humans have always moved our bodies. This natural movement, the inspiration for ESSENTRICS, is the most effective means of strengthening every muscle in the body and stopping aging in its tracks.

THE "WORKOUTS" OF THE PAST WERE THE BEST

Strong, flexible muscles are essential for every waking moment of your life. You need your arms, hands, and fingers to be strong and flexible enough so that you can open doors, carry everyday household items, put on your clothes, throw a ball with your grandchildren, reach into high cupboards, type on a computer. Muscles make it possible to complete any of the normal, everyday tasks life requires of you.

The human body has no superfluous parts. Every single part has a function and a purpose, and it is our job to maintain each part. Anything less than a full-body workout leaves the unexercised muscles vulnerable to atrophy. But research on elders has proved that exercise not only increases strength but also reduces oxidative stress and improves mitochondrial dysfunction, the two primary triggers for the aging process.[42]

If you watch children playing in a playground or park, you'll see them engaging their full bodies through a variety of movements. As they run around in a game of tag, they make rapid changes of direction to escape being caught. This naturally engages vast numbers of muscles, from the heart to the arms, hips, legs, and feet. They have to bend and rotate on the spine, as they turn their heads and twist their bodies. Tag is a wonderful activity to stimulate children's growth and muscle development. Also, remember the seesaw in the old playgrounds? What an amazing fitness apparatus it was, requiring foot, knee, and hip work as the children pumped it up and down. As a complement, the children's swing set uses the full range of motion in the shoulder joints while it is strengthening the abdominal and spinal muscles as the child leans forward and backward to generate enough momentum to propel the swing higher and higher. Young children, when given the opportunity, dynamically stretch and stimulate every muscle and joint in their bodies simply by playing.

Similarly, adult domestic chores can also work the full-body musculature, if we allow them to. Making a bed requires bending forward, which engages both the abdominal muscles and the spine. Cleaning windows works the shoulders, spine, and waist. Mopping the floor requires lifting a heavy bucket of water and lowering it to the floor, engaging the shoulders, arms, and hands. Pushing heavy objects, as when you move furniture, strengthens the hips, spine, and shoulders; and reaching to dust the top of your window frames stretches the muscles of the spine. These simple ideas engage the full body from head to toe, rebalancing and strengthening the entire musculature.

But the unfortunate truth is that many of us rarely do these chores anymore, and if we do them at all we don't do them long enough to derive any real benefit from them. The irony is that laborsaving devices have worked too well—they haven't just "saved" labor; they've actually spared most people in the Western world from having to do any labor at all. Most of us do not mop floors or push furniture on a regular basis, but once you understand the unique benefits of everyday movement for the human body, you can apply the same concepts to a workout routine.

When we string together a bunch of exercises that look like everyday activities, we are better able to work through our full-body musculature in a short time. There is actually a name for this type of movement: isotonic. I designed the exercises in ESSENTRICS to mimic daily life or familiar movements, and I then scientifically sequenced them together to stretch and strengthen all 620 muscles.

THE SCIENCE OF EVERYDAY MOVEMENTS

While these everyday movements seem simple to us, they're actually combinations of hundreds of smaller movements. For example, one of the better isotonic exercises that mimic the action of everyday life is cleaning a table, which uses your shoulder, abdominal, and back muscles and also targets your waist! Let's take a closer look at the technical terms for these movements and how they describe the process your body uses to strengthen itself.[43]

Isotonic

"Isotonic" literally means equally resistant. In exercise science, isotonic contraction is a contraction in which the tension, or resistance, remains constant as the muscle either shortens or lengthens. Lifting an object off a desk, walking, and running all involve isotonic contractions. We see isotonic exercise in the gym when a dumbbell is lifted from the ground and used to perform an exercise. The resistance (tension) generated by the dumbbell is now the constant—if you pick up a 10-pound dumbbell, it will weigh 10 pounds whatever you do with it.

In ESSENTRICS, you will not use any external weights such as dumbbells. Instead, you will use your own body mass as the constant weight. In the entire program, you are always in motion and the resistance (tension) is generated by your body, which is now the constant. If you lift your 20-pound leg, it becomes the constant—it will weigh 20 pounds whatever you do with it.

Concentric

Also referred to as positive training, concentric movement happens when the muscle shortens during tension. Concentric movement also causes a shortening of the angle of the joint. One example of a concentric movement is a biceps curl: When we lift a weight by bending the elbow, the biceps flexes and the muscle shortens.

When the muscles are challenged to any degree, they react by fighting back and strengthening. Lifting weights, running, tennis, hockey, squash, baseball, and football are all activities that concentrically strengthen the muscles, as most of the movements in these sports are done with bent joints. In these sports, the power is generated with bent knees and elbows, pulling the muscles toward the center of the body in a concentric motion. The bending of the knees and elbows in concentric movement is how the body develops bulkier muscles.

Eccentric

Eccentric movement happens when a muscle extends and lengthens while in contraction. For example, when we lower a heavy bag of groceries, the elbow straightens and makes the biceps lengthen, creating an eccentric movement. Even though it is elongating as it lowers the heavy groceries, the biceps remains contracted. Eccentric movement is also referred to as negative training.

All movement originates in protein filaments that are the building blocks of the muscles. Millions of these filaments are bundled together to make a muscle. These protein filaments slide together or apart as we strengthen or stretch them. Eccentric movement sends conflicting messages to the protein filaments. One message is to contract or slide together while the other is to lengthen or pull apart, thus creating a tug-of-war effect. That tug-of-war among the protein filaments is what creates strong and lean muscles.

In ESSENTRICS, we are always extending every movement, straightening the legs and arms and pulling away from the center as much as possible. The muscles are given two commands: one to shorten and one to lengthen, creating a tug-of-war. We all know how much effort is expended in a tug-of-war, and when people start the program their muscles often tremble. Not surprisingly, the tug-of-war within ESSENTRICS' two messages and the added stress caused by the heavier weight from a longer lever makes a beginner's muscles tremble. Often the muscles will continue to tremble until they become strong enough to support the lengthened position.

You can see the results of eccentric training by looking at a ballet dancer's body, which is famously strong, lean, and well defined. Many people come to us seeking a ballet dancer's thin, strong body, with its perfect posture. That's one of the reasons we designed this program—to help our clients achieve that look!

Clearly, eccentric exercises benefit us in multiple ways. But why are static exercises so dangerous?

HOLDING POSES HURTS US

When we move in our daily lives, we move smoothly from one activity to another. We don't stop to hold a pose; we transition seamlessly into the next movement. We are not robots and should not train ourselves to move like them, especially while doing exercises.

We should also not force ourselves to hold positions for long periods of time, which requires a great deal of strength and many hours of training to do safely and effectively. High-performance athletes and ballet dancers train for hours a day, from a very young age, to be able to hold poses properly. One of the most challenging parts in the famous ballet *Swan Lake* demands that the corps de ballet hold poses while the Swan Queen dances with the Prince. In *Swan Lake*, I would dance nonstop for three hours, but by far the most difficult part always was holding those poses!

Holding positions requires much more strength than most people realize, and can cause problematic imbalances in the rest of the body. A workout that requires such controlled pauses is great for athletes but difficult and dangerous for average people. The extreme strength required to hold a pose can place tremendous stress on the muscles, causing, or leading to, pain and injury. For example, carpal tunnel syndrome, tennis elbow, and back pain are all stress-related injuries that are very common in people who practice yoga.

The ESSENTRICS exercises are exaggerated so as to maximize benefits of the simultaneous strengthening and stretching. When the body is in continuous motion, the muscles never have a chance to seize up and compress, as they are repeatedly being stretched to their maximum. Once they reach their maximum flexibility in one movement, they continue on into the next one, never stopping. We strengthen them and simultaneously stretch them because we are always in *motion.*

All movements require some degree of strength. Even something as simple as moving your little finger requires a tiny bit of strength. A program that involves continuous motion is by definition always strengthening the muscles. Because the muscles are being stretched to their maximum in this program they are being strengthened in a lengthened or *decompressed* position. This is what eccentric movement is all about.

THE SLIDING DOOR OF STRENGTH AND FLEXIBILITY

A muscle is made up of many cells bundled together. The strength of one cell alone is insignificant, but when many tiny cells are bundled together, they become a powerful force. Each cell has stringlike fibers that slide together or apart every time we move, just as the sliding doors of a store open and close. The stringy fibers within each cell slide together when we contract our muscles and slide apart when we stretch them.

But there is a catch: The law of all movement is that muscles have to contract when we move and have to relax when the movement is finished. When the muscles contract, the fibers slide together, and when the movement is complete the muscles automatically slide apart. Like sliding doors, muscle cells have preset limits on how far they can slide in either direction. When the two sides of a sliding door move toward each other, they are stopped when they touch; they don't go past their point of contact. That's exactly the way muscle cells work: They slide until each reaches the tip of the other, and then they stop. The same principle applies when sliding doors separate: They slide neatly into a slot in the walls. Muscle cells, too, can slide apart for only a predetermined distance. If they slide beyond that point, they tear, an effect we refer to as a torn muscle.

Each muscle has the ability to slide to a predestined length; it can contract 25 percent of its resting length when it slides in and 75 percent when it slides out. Most people use only 30 to 40 percent of their muscles' ability to slide in either direction because daily life doesn't tend to require maximum use of our strength and flexibility.

In contrast, athletes, dancers, and fitness enthusiasts will use a greater range of motion in their muscles than average people. A ballerina doing splits is taking her hip mobility to its absolute extreme; a weight lifter might maximally contract his muscles as he lifts 150 pounds over his head. And while these are extreme examples, they illustrate an important lesson: In our day-to-day lives, we do not even come close to approaching the limits of what our bodies are capable of doing.

Our bodies have natural strength and a natural range of motion. To maintain our good posture, energy levels, and freedom from pain, we need to maintain, at a minimum, a 50 to 70 percent range of motion in all of our muscles. We need them to slide easily into a state of contraction or a state of flexibility. If there is no movement in the individual muscle cells, then it goes without saying that movement within the larger muscle will be impeded as well. And as we've discussed, a lack of movement leads inexorably to atrophy and cell death.

In order to slow down and reverse the aging process, we need to have both flexible and strong muscles; this means we have to do a combination of strength *and* flexibility exercises. Strengthening alone will slide the cells in only one direction, and flexibility alone will slide the cells in only the other direction. An equal combination of both dynamics, strengthening and stretching, is required to gain and maintain a sufficiently large range of motion to keep us feeling young, relaxed, and comfortable in our bodies.

THE FORCE OF GRAVITY

Another facet of aging that we must counter is the force of gravity. As we age and our cells become weaker, gravity's effects are amplified and our bodies begin to look unflatteringly saggy and soft. The force of gravity is constantly pulling us downward, but we can reverse that downward tug by consciously pulling ourselves upward, against it. Lifting our arms above our heads is one of the simplest and most effective ways to reverse the shrinking and sagging of our muscles, particularly the muscles of the spine and trunk. If we don't do this, we are likely to shrink faster than we need to.

Our 620 muscles run in many directions and patterns: vertically, horizontally, and diagonally across the body. To fight gravity, we need to pull the vertical muscles upward, as these are the main cause of our drooping and sagging. Some of the largest vertical muscles are found around our spine and trunk, so every time we lift our arms above our heads we are training those muscles to maintain their length and helping them resist gravity.

If the vertical muscles are not lengthened and strengthened to their maximum, they will shrink to the length that they are accustomed to. The human body is an efficient machine, and those cells that are left unused become tagged as unnecessary and are allowed to shrink and die. Furthermore, as muscles contract, they gradually get tighter and tighter, leading to compression of the joints. Unless we exercise our full range of motion, we leave ourselves open to poor posture, drooping shoulders, low energy levels, and even arthritis of the spine. Corrective exercise, centered on reaching toward the ceiling, prevents these negative outcomes by lengthening the spinal muscles and inhibiting atrophy.

The solution is so simple, yet most people are too focused on following a complicated exercise regimen to believe it can be this easy. Try this one exercise: Pull one arm at a time toward the ceiling for a total of 32 repetitions. Alternate arms with each reach, and do this consistently for 5 minutes every day. It will make you look and feel younger, and it should rapidly improve your posture.

OTHER FITNESS OPTIONS

When it comes to other sports or fitness programs, very few programs rebalance all 620 muscles and protect the joints. That is why I created ESSENTRICS. My first love was tai chi, which is also a full-body movement technique. But if I missed a session (as I often did, owing to my hectic schedule), I found it difficult to reintegrate myself into the group because the routines changed a little bit with every class. I wanted to create a program that would be as enjoyable as tai chi but that anyone could follow easily; those goals helped inspire this program.

Many people love activities like walking, running, weight training, yoga, Pilates, skiing, swimming, and tennis. All of these activities are fun to do, but every one of them is known to damage the joints, unbalance the muscles, cause chronic pain, and not use all 620 muscles.

My suggestion to you: If you love it, do it. Just be smart about using all of your muscles over the course of your day, both with everyday motions and with regular rebalancing training.

POWER AND ENDURANCE

Nothing signifies old age quite so aptly as someone whose every movement is laborious, someone for whom even routine tasks take forever to accomplish. Anyone who is used to moving quickly knows it is a lesson in patience to be around someone who takes forever clearing dishes off a table, walking up the stairs, getting up from a sofa, or getting out of a car. Slowing down is a natural sign of aging, but premature slowing down is not, and can be easily reversed.

What causes us to slow down and have trouble doing simple tasks is a lack of strength, which has two components: power and endurance. We need them both to be able to do life's daily tasks with ease and comfort. Power is measured by the ability to lift a heavy object and endurance is measured by the ability to keep moving for long periods of time. Power gives us the ability to lift heavy items or simply lift our own body off the sofa easily. Endurance allows us to run marathons, take long hikes, or simply walk for more than five minutes without tiring.

Gaining power and endurance can be accomplished with relative ease and speed, and at any age. Both power and endurance are in the "strength family," where improvement requires us to do strengthening exercises. The power required to lift a heavy bag of groceries isn't the same as the power required of a professional baseball player to hit a home run. Nor is the endurance required to carry the groceries from the store to your car in the parking lot the same endurance required of a marathon runner. But the basic principles are the same. You do not need to train with the intensity of these athletes to develop the power and endurance necessary to lead a normal, active life. Instead, you need to align your training habits with your goals.

Power requires immediate explosive strength, whereas endurance requires effort sustained over a length of time. Strong muscles are required for both power and strength, but we use a different approach to train for each one. Power is developed by doing repetitive movements using the weight of the entire body. Power movements are those rapid movements requiring a sudden burst of strength; activities such as skiing, tennis, golf, and carpentry all require different degrees of power. Some of these activities might also require endurance, if we prolong them.

Endurance is the ability to keep moving for an extended period of time without tiring. Endurance activities are slow and steady, and we undertake them for more than five minutes. In addition to running races, cycling for several miles, and swimming many laps, these include cutting grass, weeding, vacuuming, painting walls, and going for long walks.

One of the greatest difficulties of aging is that we fail to perceive our gradual loss of strength and flexibility; we are made aware of it only when we wake up one painful morning to discover that what was once second nature now requires strenuous effort. The contrast is most evident when we are around young people, who seem to brim with energy. But the speed of the young is also just a product of explosive power and endurance strength. Young people have these attributes naturally; as we get older, we have to work for them!

As we age, we subconsciously let ourselves take smaller, slower strides. In order to reverse this part of the aging process, and increase both power and endurance, we have to consciously take wider, larger strides and move faster when we walk. This wider, faster stride will increase our explosive power. If we walk rapidly for at least 20 minutes every day, we will have strengthened the endurance and power of our lower body (hips, knees, and feet) immensely. In addition to taking wider strides, try moving faster in everything you do. Turn your daily tasks into antiaging workouts—move rapidly and make yourself do bigger, rather than smaller, movements.

Public attitudes toward smoking have changed dramatically in the last twenty years. Millions of people quit smoking once they were shown how bad cigarettes were for their health. I believe that people who genuinely understand the relationship between regular, full-body exercise, their health, and their ability to look and feel young well into their senior years will take this information and radically change the way they live. No one wants to age and no one wants to age rapidly. The price—from chronic pain to the loss of independence and the attendant emotional distress—is simply too high.

Until now, we didn't know how to stop the effects of aging, but now that I know the science behind aging, I never miss a single day of giving my body 20 to 30 minutes of full-body exercising. This method not only helps reverse the aging process but also helps us to avoid diseases and conditions that can severely reduce our quality of life.

CHAPTER 7

GET MOVING

THE CONNECTION BETWEEN FITNESS AND DISEASE PREVENTION

We've talked about how ESSENTRICS protects against muscle loss and how our muscles keep us young. Now let's talk about how powerfully muscles can care for the rest of the body.

Another myth of aging that people blithely accept is that we're all going to get sick at some point—that disease goes hand in hand with aging. Not true. Many diet and lifestyle factors can help you prevent the onset of disease, and one of the most powerful is the ability of exercise to build muscle. Fitness can not only help you lose weight and have more energy but also keep you disease-free. We'll look at how the strength of your muscles affects the other systems in your body—such as the cardiovascular, digestive, and neurological systems. These can get weaker with age, but don't have to if you commit to exercise.

The body is like a complex car that has different systems; all have to be in good working order or the car won't run. The wheels are like the muscles, the engine is like the cardiovascular system, the transmission and brakes are like the nervous system, and the burning of gas is like the digestive system. If one of those parts isn't working the car won't go. Or if the parts are rusted and worn out, then the car might run, but badly.

This is where healthy strong flexible muscles come in. The role of the muscles is to keep the systems healthy; to assist the cardiovascular system in the distribution of blood into every cell of the body; to cleanse out toxins that damage the organs; to assist the digestive system in flushing out waste products; and much more. Without strong active healthy muscles working in harmony with them, the systems become exhausted and break down prematurely. When this happens we feel and look unhealthy, we become prone to getting sick, and we take much longer than necessary to recover.

Strong flexible muscles keep you healthy, and when you do get sick, they help you to recover rapidly and fully! With regard to your desire to remain young and vibrant the muscular system is the most important system in your body. When you let your muscular system become weak, all the other systems that keep you alive are directly affected. Without strong flexible muscles all the other systems will age rapidly through overuse and decay. One Danish study looked at the impact of smoking tobacco, high alcohol consumption, physical inactivity, and overweight on expected lifetime. The researchers combined life tables and disease prevalence data from over 14,000 participants in the Danish Health Interview Survey. They found that, on average, physically inactive people will have a life span that is 5 to 8 years shorter than that of physically active people.[44]

We know that if we don't exercise all 620 muscles, they will atrophy. When this happens, we will find it much more difficult to maintain our health because with atrophy comes a deterioration of the systems of the body required to keep us healthy.

CARDIOVASCULAR SYSTEM

The heart is our most important muscle; we must protect it at all costs. The muscular system has a very important role to play in keeping the cardiovascular system fit and functioning at full capability. The muscular system is designed to work in harmony with the heart, veins, and arteries, helping to improve circulation and reducing some of our cardiovascular workload. When the heart's workload is reduced, wear and tear on important parts of the cardiovascular system is reduced, and damage that can trigger inflammation and heart disease is prevented.

Muscles have a direct role in the efficiency of the circulation of blood throughout our bodies. Active muscles are designed to perform as pumps, helping the blood circulate. The pumping action of the muscles takes some of the load off the vessels, which otherwise would have to do all the pumping and delivery of blood alone. When the vessels have to do the pumping by themselves, they cannot do as effective a job as when the muscles are helping them. This means that some cells are not receiving nutrient- and oxygen-loaded blood, and so we are prone to illness and chronic tiredness—the feeling that we are dragging all day and can never get caught up on sleep. Sound familiar?

First and foremost, we need active muscles delivering nutrients and removing waste products to help us stay young. The circulatory system is the system that delivers blood to the entire body—as I sometimes say, "from brain to brawn." The circulatory system delivers nutrient-loaded oxygen-rich blood to every cell in the body and, on its return journey, acts as a garbage removal system, retrieving dead cells, toxins, and waste products. A slow sluggish circulatory system means that our cells are not receiving life-giving nutrients, nor are the poisonous toxins being flushed out of our system. This leaves us feeling and *looking* exhausted: Dull, lifeless skin is a giveaway for a sluggish circulatory system.

Recent research reported in the *New York Times* found that this cleansing effect is not the only reason our skin looks so great when we exercise. The preliminary study from researchers at McMaster University in Ontario, presented in 2014 at the annual meeting of the American Medical Society for Sports Medicine, followed a group of sedentary men and women over 65 to study the effect their exercise habits had on their skin. The researchers had this formerly sedentary group work out vigorously (at 65 percent of the subjects' maximum heart rate) for 30 minutes twice a week for 3 months. When the researchers analyzed biopsies from the subjects' skin, they discovered that the skin had changed dramatically, and more closely resembled that of people in their twenties. The researchers believe that exercise triggers the release of myokines, a type of protein released by the muscle; the myokines would travel from the muscle through the bloodstream and initiate changes in cells far away from the cells where they were released. The skin samples indicated that the levels of myokines actually leaped up by 50 percent after the start of the study.[45] Exercisers were being changed on a genetic level, and those changes were manifesting themselves in younger, dewier, less lined skin.

No face creams can replace the vibrancy that good circulation gives to the skin. No massages or facials are as powerful in cleansing and nourishing the skin as full-body circulation. I love my creams, facials, and massages, but there is nothing as effective as a good full-body workout to make your skin glow!

All we need to do is 10 minutes of large body movements every day to increase the blood flow, flush out the toxins, and inject the entire body with energy-giving oxygen and nutrients. Nothing makes us more exhausted than sitting around all day! Anyone who works in an office will attest to that. And nothing brings the sparkle back into our eyes better than a few minutes of exercise.

Large full-body movements like the ones in Classical Stretch, ESSENTRICS, and tai chi all strengthen the muscles of the cardiovascular system and facilitate the circulation of blood without any impact on the joints and provide an effective alternative to the traditional cardio workouts on the market. When the circulatory system is functioning well, we have more energy. Our brains receive more oxygen, so we think more clearly. We simply *feel better* in every way.

The Harvard school of medicine has done many studies of the health benefits of tai chi. Interestingly, the citizens of China have been doing tai chi for centuries and many remain free of exercise-related injuries for most of their lives. To this day in China you will see people doing tai chi in parks, at their workplaces, and in various public places. The Chinese are known for their longevity and good health, which can be attributed in large part to their practice of tai chi.

Furthermore, the results of studies such as those by the Harvard Medical School on tai chi showed that tai chi–type movements are valuable in preventing coronary artery disease and had an effect on various factors associated with the disease, such as lowered blood pressure, a boost in exercise capacity, and improved cholesterol levels. Especially given that the leading cause of death in America is coronary artery disease, this finding has very important implications.[46]

With their large sweeping muscle movements, these exercise programs relieve the strain on the arteries caused by a buildup of plaque in artery walls. Muscle movement involves contraction and relaxation, a pumping motion that acts to assist the circulation of blood into the extremities and back to the heart. Large muscle movements act as a partner to the heart muscle in the circulation of blood, taking the overload off the heart and distributing the effort of full circulation. One review of tai chi's effectiveness in preventing chronic heart disease, completed for *Cochrane Database Systemic Reviews*, reported that six studies had found tai chi reduced participants' systolic blood pressure by up to 22 points and three studies had found it reduced diastolic blood pressure by as much as 12 points.[47] Two studies also found reductions in total cholesterol, LDL-C, and triglycerides. Clearly, there's a compelling cardiovascular rationale for the ancient practice of tai chi and similar approaches, such as ESSENTRICS.

I personally don't enjoy traditional cardio workouts such as aerobics or running on a treadmill, so I have sought to find alternatives. If you do enjoy them, don't stop doing them, but these high-impact forms of exercise have proved to damage joints if they are done over many years. I have many clients who love running and want to continue running all their lives. You should be able to do so; you just need to protect your joints with correct strengthening and simultaneous stretching exercises. Unfortunately, very few runners take the time to protect their joints. I've worked with many runners over 45 who have been forced to stop running because of joint pain or damage. No one should have to stop doing a favorite sport, especially if it is beneficial to the cardiovascular system or other body systems, but athletes must protect their joints with preventive exercises so that the joints will last a lifetime.

DIGESTIVE SYSTEM

The digestive system is designed to take the food we eat and break it into molecules small enough to be absorbed through the walls of our cells and burned as fuel in our mitochondria, the calorie-burning furnaces of our cells. Digestion is achieved through a complex system of tubing (the esophagus and intestines) and chemical processing stations (liver, pancreas, kidneys, and bladder). The system starts in the mouth and ends when the nutrients get delivered to cells, excess fat gets delivered to fat storage units, and waste products get eliminated.

When everything is running smoothly, we should be totally unaware that within the walls of the body this amazing feat is being accomplished. We should feel no pain or discomfort or bloating as the food makes its way through the system.

The digestive system is housed in the torso. Every human being is born with sufficient space for the digestive system to function efficiently. The catch is that we have enough space only if we have good posture, when our spine is at its longest. Poor posture collapses the spine and shortens the space required to comfortably house the digestive system. The result is that the tubes and organs become compressed and push outward against the walls of the body. You cannot squish the tubes and factories by limiting their space and still expect them to function effortlessly. This reduction of space makes the passage of the food uncomfortable, inefficient, and painful.

It doesn't take a scientific study to show us that many Americans have a big problem with digestive discomfort. Anyone who walks down the aisles of a pharmacy will be confronted by row upon row of over-the-counter digestive medications.

Two parts of the digestive system can be helped with exercise:

1. the upper part, where problems such as heartburn, acid reflux, and choking can occur

2. the lower part, where issues such as constipation and poor elimination are common

The upper part, the area of the body from the waist up, is most affected by poor posture as the spine droops forward, collapsing the rib cage and shrinking our height. When the body droops forward, the rib cage has to go somewhere, and that is how the esophagus tubing gets blocked. The only place that the ribs can go is backward toward your spine, which means the lungs, esophagus, heart, and liver are all crammed inside and fighting for space by pushing against one another. While all the crowding is happening inside your rib cage area, the food you have just eaten is trying to make its way into your stomach. Simply straightening your posture makes digestion easier and more comfortable.

Good posture is achieved by lengthening and strengthening all the muscles of the torso. Many people don't know how to improve their posture and so they get very discouraged. In Part III, I will share a series of simple exercises to show you how to improve your posture. (It's easier than you think!)

The second part of the digestive system that requires strong muscles is the intestinal part, which most people refer to as the stomach. When we think our "stomach" is bloated, it is probably not our stomach at all but our intestines.

The intestines are a 30-foot-long hose or tube that occupies the space between the waist and rectum. The intestines are lined with a type of muscle that involuntarily pushes the feces through without our having to think about it. Without these involuntary muscles, the feces would be incapable of moving through the intestines. Like other "in-groups" of muscles that work as assistants to certain groups of muscles, the abdominal muscles are designed to act in partnership with the intestinal muscles: they help the intestinal muscles push the feces through the intestines.

If we lead a sedentary life, we will have weak abdominal muscles. The intestinal muscles won't have anything to push against, and that lack will slow down the movement of feces through our intestines, leading to a hardening of the feces and constipation.

When we see people who have a large protruding abdomen we say they have a "big stomach," but what is really happening is that they have weak abdominal muscles so their intestines are hanging out! When the abdominal muscles are weak there is nothing keeping the intestines in place, so—to repeat—they hang out.

Think of the "toothpaste effect": The more we twist and squeeze our toothpaste tube, the easier it is to squeeze the toothpaste out. Our intestines are tubes and they need all the help we can give them to make elimination fast and pain-free. Relaxed, easy movements that involve twisting and turning and as much movement of the torso as possible loosen up the "innards," helping encourage easy elimination.

THE NEUROLOGICAL SYSTEM

The neurological system, which is made up of the brain and nerves, is a sending-and-receiving system that communicates with every cell of the body. The neurological system is the command center responsible for regulating every part of the body—from heating and cooling to healing and nourishing to simply helping us experience, understand, and enjoy our lives. And a recent explosion of research has found that exercise is by far the best medicine to protect and support the function of your neurological system, especially your brain.

Exercise is a proven antidepressant; exercise helps us relax, focus, concentrate—and come up with great ideas. Exercise even increases the size of our brains. By raising our levels of BDNF—brain-derived neurotrophic factor, sometimes called "MiracleGro for the brain"—exercise causes the stem cells in our brain to create new neurons and greatly increases the number and function of mitochondria in our brain cells. What could be better than more energy factories in our brains?[48]

In younger adults, exercise-induced brain growth takes place mainly in our hippocampus, the primary site of memory in the brain, and this growth may help prevent the onset (or slow the development) of cognitive decline and Alzheimer's disease. This effect is even more important among older adults, especially those at highest risk. One study conducted by the Cleveland Clinic followed 97 older folks (ages 65 to 89) who had not yet shown signs of cognitive decline. After 18 months they found that those at highest genetic risk for Alzheimer's disease who didn't exercise had lost 3 percent of their brain mass in those 18 months, while those at high risk who had exercised lost no brain mass at all.[49]

Another neurological concern as we grow older is trouble maintaining our balance—truly one of the most frightening signs of aging. If we don't feel steady on our feet, ordinary activities—walking to our car, taking a bus, visiting friends—become daunting challenges with the potential for serious injury. Add to that the sense that you are "losing it," and neurological concerns can be terrifying.

Fear of falling is a real and all too common concern in old age, one that makes us feel dependent on others as we develop a growing feeling of insecurity about our safety. The solution is to start taking precautions against losing balance before we age! The loss of balance does not happen rapidly; the nerves that communicate with our muscles and keep us steady take decades to age and die.

We need something called balance reflexes to fire a message into our muscles when we are in danger of losing our balance. The loss of balance reflexes is generally a case of simple neglect, a failure on our part to stimulate these reflexes when we still have them. As with every other part of our body, the maxim "Use it or lose it" is applicable: It is within our power to prevent, delay, minimize, or reverse the symptoms of poor balance.

All movement—from sitting on a chair to standing and walking—requires us to stay on balance. Without balance reflexes, we would be incapable of doing any of the above movements. Being on balance is basic to human life and it works when the brain sends messages to fire up the appropriate muscles to prevent us from falling over. A baby learns to sit without falling by slowly stimulating its balance reflexes through trial and error. Every time it falls over, the baby's balance reflexes are stimulated until eventually the balance reflexes and muscles become sufficiently strong to keep the infant on balance.

As we age, the reverse happens: When we lose our balance or feel unsteady, we instinctively reach for a railing or another person, or anything to prevent us from falling. But the result is that we are robbed of opportunities to stimulate our balance reflexes, and so they shrivel up and atrophy, compounding our balance troubles rather than solving them.

In our day-to-day lives, we rarely put ourselves in dangerous, off-balance situations. We subconsciously sense when we are about to lose our balance and take instant precautions to regain it, as when we slow our pace before walking over a patch of ice. It is important to note that when we strengthen our muscles, we do not automatically strengthen our balance reflexes. The small, subconscious acts we take to stabilize ourselves before we lose our balance also prevent us from stimulating our balance reflexes and set us up for long-term degeneration of those reflexes.

The trouble is that most people do not understand the importance of exercising the balance reflexes. As children, all of us ran, jumped, crawled, and did cartwheels or other forms of gymnastics. We were unwittingly exercising our balance reflexes and reinforcing the importance of these connections in our brain. As we mature, however, and take on the responsibilities of adulthood, most people become sedentary, letting the vital neurological connections they've built in their youth begin to disintegrate. Rather than seek out unstable situations, we subconsciously avoid them; we use a walking stick or grab the railing on stairs out of a sense of precaution rather than necessity.

When we are young, our nerve fibers can grow an inch a year, but after a certain age they cannot. This is why we have to do all we can to maintain whatever balance reflexes we have to prevent any further atrophy and death of nerve cells. Once dead, they are gone forever. Whatever the state of your balance reflexes is today, start challenging them now in order to prevent any further loss of nerve cells. (See "Exercises to Stimulate the Neurological System" (page 102) for some fast and simple exercises that you can do anywhere.)

Different health problems connected to aging have a way of creeping up on us. At first, we are completely unaware that we lean on a wall for support or sit on a chair to take off our shoes or hold the arm of a chair to help us sit down or stand up. Simple exercises like standing on one leg and not holding a support while writing the alphabet with the other leg will really help prevent any further loss of the valuable nerves called balance reflexes. It is never too late to start!

In addition to stimulating the balance reflexes, the neurological system plays thousands of other vital roles in keeping us feeling young, healthy, and active. The foremost concern for most of us as we head into our senior years is remaining lucid and mentally focused by maintaining as many brain cells as possible. I am always interested in any studies that offer helpful tips on how to keep the brain functioning optimally.

Scientists know that aerobic exercise increases memory and brain capacity, and in recent years it has been established that the same theory applies for less strenuous types of exercise such as tai chi. According to scientists from the University of South Florida and Fudan University, when a group of non-senile elders from China participated in

EXERCISES TO STIMULATE
THE NEUROLOGICAL SYSTEM

In everyday life, we never deliberately put ourselves in off-balance situations, but we need to exercise the balance reflexes in order to prevent atrophy.

ABC Exercise: One easy way of stimulating your balance reflexes is standing on one leg while "writing" the alphabet with your other leg (don't hold on to anything for support). You will probably wobble and struggle to stay on balance, but the effort will stimulate your reflexes. Try to make it through the entire alphabet before changing legs. Writing the alphabet can be done every day until you can write the entire alphabet; then do it at least three times a week just to keep the reflexes from atrophying.

Commuter's Exercise: Challenge yourself to stand tall without using the handholds on the bus or train. Be prepared to grab hold if you must, but the instability created by the motion of the vehicle provides an excellent challenge for the tiny fibers of your balance reflexes.

Yoga: Yoga offers many poses that force the participant to stand on one leg or in positions of instability. The more you wobble around doing a pose, the better stimulation your balance reflexes receive. Doing yoga on a regular basis will strengthen the neurological connections to the muscles—just be sure to balance it out with ESSENTRICS exercises so you don't overtrain your muscles. Overtraining could lead to imbalances.

As much as possible, we should not shy away from these opportunities to test ourselves. When walking up and down stairs, or getting dressed, or putting on shoes, do your best to maintain your own balance without reaching for a chair or wall.

low-intensity exercise such as tai chi three times a week, compared with those who did not, subjects experienced an increase in brain volume, enhanced memory, and improved cognitive abilities.[50] As dementia is linked to brain shrinkage, it can be assumed that low-intensity physical activity such as tai chi or ESSENTRICS can delay symptoms of dementia.[51]

Once again, I am impressed that the body has included in its self-healing systems a process to keep brain cells alive as long as possible. And once again it seems that moving our muscles is part of the process of maintaining life—even brain-cell life!

As I continued to develop the ESSENTRICS technique, I adopted many of the principles of tai chi and incorporated them into my program. The most obvious element of tai chi that inspired me is sweeping, full-body, rotational movement. I designed similar movements and made them easy to follow and safe for anyone to do, at no matter what age or level of fitness. Through my extensive experience and time teaching my technique, I have come to see that participants who do ESSENTRICS will be likely to reap neurological, cardiovascular, and digestive benefits similar to those of tai chi—a fact that makes me immensely proud.

CHAPTER 8

PREVENT AND HEAL AFTER INJURY

When the wheels of a car are off balance, the car pulls dangerously to one side; this effect makes the car accident-prone and causes unnecessary wear and tear on the entire vehicle. Driving an unbalanced car is a dangerous, awkward, and unpleasant experience—so we tend to fix it right away. Unfortunately, we are rarely as attentive when it comes to our bodies.

When we have minor injuries or aches and pains, most of us tend to ignore the discomfort. Eventually we may come to tolerate a great deal of pain, hoping it will disappear on its own, or we may simply accept is as a part of life. Exercising to treat the pain is not a commonly prescribed approach, and its effectiveness and efficiency are vastly underestimated.

Rebalancing the body is similar to rebalancing the wheels of a car: All four wheels need to be balanced in relation to one another for proper function. You can't adjust one wheel and hope the other wheels will fall naturally into place. Pinpointing one muscle group and ignoring the others will not eliminate a problem.

Focused, thorough work is necessary to resolve an imbalance, but once the issue has been addressed, the pain is often alleviated. As with a car, however, proper care and maintenance are essential! We can't expect the body to remain eternally "fixed"; once we've rebalanced, the body is in constant need of tweaks and adjustments in order to heal and prevent injuries. A consistent practice of ESSENTRICS accomplishes both of these goals.

HEALING AFTER INJURY

The World Health Organization defines health as "a state of complete physical, mental, and social well-being and not merely the absence of disease or infirmity."[52] Fitness and exercise are now recognized as essential to the achievement of good health and healing. In order for exercise to facilitate the healing process, several basic criteria must be met:

1. The program must not cause further damage or injury.

2. Blood flow must be brought into the afflicted area.

3. The injured area must be rebalanced.

4. The muscles must be returned to their natural level of strength and flexibility.

5. The entire body must be engaged so as not to cause further imbalance.

As a full-body strengthening and rebalancing fitness and flexibility program, ESSENTRICS meets all these basic criteria.

My program has been used to heal many common, chronic conditions such as back pain, osteoporosis, fibromyalgia, arthritis, frozen shoulder, and knee and hip pain. Movement is a natural part of all healing and should not be dismissed as optional. The right movements can increase the rate of healing as well as prevent many aches and pains in the first place.

(One important note: Even though I have had the honor of relieving many people of chronic pain and injury, I don't want to overstate my credentials. I am not a medical practitioner or doctor. I do not want to mislead anyone by exaggerating what correct exercise can do to help. Grave illness or disease is not something that exercise has the ability to cure. If you are in constant pain or you are recovering from a major injury or surgery, I always recommend that you get a doctor's or physiotherapist's permission before beginning an exercise regimen.)

HEALING AND BLOOD FLOW

I often have clients who are either recovering from an injury or suffering from chronic pain. The way I approach a workout for an injured client is very different from the way I approach it for a healthy one. Strengthening and conditioning are great for healthy bodies—but not fragile bodies. When I work with healthy clients, I check first to be sure that they are in reasonably good physical shape and will benefit from the dynamics of a conditioning routine.

The word "rehabilitation" means the restoration of good health and the resumption of normal functioning. The word "conditioning" refers to challenging or stressing something in order to strengthen it. The approach to the workout that is appropriate for healthy people is at the opposite end of the fitness spectrum from the approach for injured people. One group needs vigorous conditioning and the other requires gentle rehabilitation.

While you are healing, your body is more fragile and has self-protective mechanisms that block any possible danger of reinjuring itself. After you've suffered an injury, your muscles should *not* be challenged. We have to temporarily forget about getting into shape, which can come once we have healed. The goal of any exercise is to increase the rate of healing.

At first glance, the ESSENTRICS healing workouts might seem similar to conditioning workouts, as we are using many of the same movements, exercises, and techniques. However, upon examining both types of workouts, you will notice that the conditioning routines challenge the muscles while the rehabilitation routines focus on blood circulation and relaxation.

Maximum blood circulation keeps injured tissues well fed and oxygenated. On its way out of the heart, blood is the carrier of all the healing nutrients; on its return journey, blood acts as the garbage removal system. To ease circulation and encourage blood flow, we simply have to relax our muscles as much as possible and move through the exercises like a rag doll, while breathing deeply. Years of experience working with injured people has taught me that the more the clients relax in a workout, the faster they heal. This consistent, gentle movement is all that is required in the healing phase of rehabilitation.

I have seen both personal trainers and clients become so frustrated by tight muscles that they stretch aggressively in a vain attempt to force the tightness to loosen up. But the body has natural defenses aimed at protecting the muscles against further injury. You often end up with the opposite effect: The reflexes go into protection mode, making the muscles even tighter and more contracted, and the injury is worsened rather than healed. Strength training, which is supposed to increase power in healthy muscles, has the opposite effect when used on injured muscles.

To speed healing, you can also use another very important trick: avoidance. For example, if you have an injured knee, you work every group of muscles in the body *except* the knee. You relax the injured knee while gently stretching and strengthening the ankles, calves, quadriceps, inner and outer thighs, hamstrings, gluteus group, and so on, working every muscle except the knee itself. Not going near the injury while releasing tension in all the peripheral muscles has the effect of taking the strain off the injured area. Doing a full-body workout is the most effective way to heal a local area, as long as you keep the injured area relaxed.

The amazing thing is that you can do ESSENTRICS even when you are injured. Often, students will join a group class when they are suffering from some minor pain or injury and they have no problem participating in class as long as they do the workout in "relaxed healing mode." At the start of the class, I remind them, "Anyone who is injured, just do the same workout—but be lazy in your execution."

Once you have a doctor's permission, I encourage you to exercise when you are in rehabilitation—but be sure to carefully monitor yourself to make sure you are *not working*. You will recover far more rapidly if you don't put any effort into the movements. If you're used to thinking of exercise as a means of getting into shape, you may resist the idea of being told to be lazy. But trust me: After doing one workout like a rag doll, you'll change your tune. Most of my injured students smile with relief—they tell me they feel better and are actually capable of moving more freely than they were prior to the class. To me this is the magic of the human body: Your body knows how to protect itself and how to heal.

HEALING GLOBALLY *IS* HEALING LOCALLY

Injuries are never local and the healing of injuries should not be local either. To prevent injuries, all 620 muscles in the body must be equally flexible and strong. To heal injuries, the injured muscles must be returned to an equal balance of strength and flexibility with the rest of the body.

THE ROLE OF AWARENESS IN INJURY PREVENTION

A major part of injury prevention is awareness, the link between the mind and the body. Awareness in ESSENTRICS is the conscious and deliberate alignment of all joints: knees, hips, and spine. Awareness is being sensitive to when a movement feels wrong, feels awkward, or is putting an unhealthy strain on muscles. The more aware you are, the better any movement is performed, and the better the results will be.

Body awareness is the integration of several objectives into one. First, you develop an awareness of your body and its movements, which helps you strengthen the muscles to support and correct the change. In ballet and modern dance, students are trained to know exactly which muscles to use in order to execute a movement. But this awareness does not come naturally to most people. Without dance training, many people have trouble isolating specific muscles, which I believe is critical to staying safe and getting the maximum benefits of any fitness program.

In fact, most people are unaware of how they move in most everyday activities, such as sitting, standing, or walking. Regardless of whether we are conscious of them or not, these movements actively train the body—correctly or incorrectly. Poor posture is an example. Habitual poor posture develops the muscles accordingly—the pectorals begin to shrink, the back muscles weaken, the shoulders round, and the neck becomes overstretched. Many people's body awareness is so poor that they can stand with poor posture feeling as though they are standing correctly. It's only when they see themselves in a mirror that they realize how bad their posture actually is.

When someone becomes accustomed to poor posture, correct posture feels uncomfortable and wrong. You will need time to reprogram your mind and strengthen your muscles to achieve good posture and feel comfortable with it. During the transition period from bad to good posture, you have to be motivated and committed to making the change or you will quickly revert to bad posture.

The benefits of using your awareness to correct a lifetime of bad habits (bad posture, heavy walk, or any other mechanical action that can lead to injury) cannot be overstated—you will easily develop a more attractive body, or attain greater success as an athlete, or simply learn to appreciate the power and the glory of your own body, no matter how old you are.[53]

Injuries may seem local, but often the actual damage or trauma may be caused by tension or weakness in another part of the muscle chain to which the injured muscles are attached. For example, a knee injury could be caused by tightness in the hamstrings or calves. Back pain could be caused by tight hamstrings, and neck pain could be caused by atrophy in the feet.

When someone has tight or overbuilt muscles, tension is created in the muscle chain and pulls on all the muscles along that chain. The extreme tension leads to a tearing of the most vulnerable muscle along the chain. The injury is caused by a chain reaction, but the initial tension might be somewhere else in the body.

The number one way to prevent injuries is to keep the full-body muscles equally strong and flexible. When people do a lot of strengthening and very little to no dynamic stretching, you will find muscle tears, sprains, and injuries. If you have tight or overbuilt muscles, your entire body is an accident waiting to happen.

Athletes often suffer from muscle tears and injuries. I'm not talking about athletes bashing into one another and getting injured—I'm talking about injuries resulting from just doing a noncombat movement in a sport. Injuries from overbuilt muscles are also very common in the aerobics and running worlds, when muscles become so tight from years of impact that the body cannot sustain the tension. Something has to give and usually does. It could be a back, groin, calf, shin, Achilles tendon, or hip— somewhere along the chain of muscles, the tension builds until the weakest point gives out.

DON'T BABY THE INJURY

Overbuilding and too much tension in the muscles are the main causes of injuries and pain. But after the injuries have healed and it is time to rebuild the body, many people make the mistake of overprotecting the previously injured area. This leads us to the next problem: atrophy.

People often make the mistake of protecting or isolating a previously injured area by depending on braces, orthotics, or bandages while training the noninjured part. Whenever a muscle is restricted from movement, it will inevitably weaken and atrophy from lack of use. Being overprotective of the original injury virtually guarantees that you will develop a chronic lifelong weakness in the area instead of just recovering from something that hurt you once and then was gone from your memory!

THE 20 PERCENT RULE

Athletes get much more out of ESSENTRICS than just increasing their flexibility. The workouts cover a broad spectrum of techniques and objectives that athletes need, from active, ballistic, and eccentric stretching to alignment, injury prevention, and body awareness. To get the best results, I always recommend the 20 percent formula: Athletes should devote 20 percent (one-fifth) of their total training time to ESSENTRICS. In practical terms, that means an athlete who does 20 hours of training weekly should put aside four of those hours to do this program. Or an amateur athlete who does five hours a week should put aside one hour for it. Athletes who follow this formula have consistently experienced fewer injuries and much improved performance.

Most athletes assume that a stretch program is solely intended to improve flexibility—so their logical question is "Why should I do it if I don't *need* flexibility?" Who doesn't need flexibility? In my experience, these same athletes often have a grocery list of aches, pains, and injuries!

Ultimately, all sports require speed, and locked joints restrict speed. Even the smallest degree of added flexibility can help any athlete increase his or her speed—every little bit brings athletes closer to the podium!

Over the years I have seen this temptation to overprotect our weakest muscles in the healing processes of everyone from injured athletes to people with congenital diseases. Both groups, in my opinion, are overly dependent on braces, orthotics, or other athletic "support" devices, which keep their injured areas weak. While these types of support can be beneficial in preventing further injury, I believe they should be used as little as possible, because the more we depend on them, the weaker the muscles become. Muscles need to be moved and engaged to gain strength, and as long as they are being restricted from movement, they cannot strengthen.

When I first suggested to Robert, a teenage client of mine who suffers from a condition associated with cerebral palsy called triplegia, that he stop using the braces on his legs, his family viewed my advice with some skepticism. He was then 15, and he had been using leg braces since birth. His doctors had said they could no longer do anything for him. In desperation, his parents turned to me. I will be totally honest: I know nothing about triplegia or how to treat it. But I do know a lot about the nature of muscles and atrophy.

When I first met him, he couldn't walk up the stairs to my studio; he was always falling down. His parents and four siblings were his constant caregivers, picking him up and helping him maneuver around their home. I gave him some basic exercises to do but the most important advice was to take off the braces as much as possible.

The next year when Robert returned, he was able to walk up the stairs on his own and stand by himself without falling down. A year after that, at Robert's annual hospital visit, the size of his calf muscle had grown by three-quarters of an inch! Needless to say, he and his family were beaming with pride. Robert and I continue to work together, each year adding more complex exercises. We have even done the fox-trot together!

Not fully rehabilitating is a mistake that many injured people make. Previously injured muscles get weaker from lack of use, so the problem is aggravated by atrophy and an imbalance. This leads to a lifetime of pain. I can't tell you how often I hear people talk about childhood injuries that are still causing pain 50 years later.

HEALING AN INJURY

We need to keep the pace of rehabilitation slow enough that the muscles surrounding the injury don't need to learn new tricks. In time, the injured muscles will heal and strengthen, picking up where they left off.

Injuries are, by definition, points of weakness, and there is a natural temptation to continue to protect these weaker body parts so as not to cause more damage. A fear of reinjury becomes a psychological challenge in the healing process. Favoring the healthier, stronger muscles is always easier than using the weak ones, but that is a common and dangerous mistake. Let's review the steps in healing:

Step 1: In pain, relax

The more relaxed your muscles are while you are exercising, the more rapidly you will heal. This is true for two reasons: Relaxation helps increase circulation and relaxation does not trigger the protective reflexes that seize the muscles and stop them from moving. Stay relaxed while exercising until the pain has totally gone away.

THE HEALING FORMULA: 10 TIPS FOR RAPID HEALING

When you are healing:

1. Focus on increasing blood flow to the entire body in order to bring healing nutrients to the injured areas.

2. The muscles need to be relaxed the entire time you are exercising. While it may take several days or several weeks, please wait until the pain goes away before changing from healing mode to training mode.

3. Never go to the end of a movement; always hold back from going to your limits.

4. Movements should be small, not large.

5. Use circular movements.

6. Work slowly.

7. Work in a "lazy" manner.

8. Always do a full-body workout.

9. Breathe deeply throughout the workout.

10. *Do not* focus on the injured muscles more than any other muscle group.

Injured muscles need the natural healing medication carried in blood cells. Blood cannot flow as effectively into contracted muscles as it does into relaxed ones. So stay relaxed if you want to heal quickly!

If you have a type A personality, you might find it frustrating to be forced to slow down and relax while exercising. Don't look upon it as exercising; tell yourself that you are doing therapeutic movements.

Step 2: Once the pain is gone, it's time to strengthen your muscles

Once the pain is gone, you can start to rebuild your muscles' strength and dynamic flexibility. Slowly increase the intensity of your workouts one day at a time. This step doesn't take long—muscles are designed to be strong and flexible.

However, be careful not to overexert them: Overexertion can reinflame the injury. When weak, injured muscles are challenged before they are fully recovered, protective reflexes kick in and block any advancement. You don't want to teach the muscles the wrong lessons. Rebuilding injured muscles to their original size and strength takes time, depending on the severity of the injury.

During the rebuilding process, don't focus too narrowly on the injured muscle. Owing to the injury, the muscles will have shrunk. If the injured area has been restricted in a cast or binding, you will also have some degree of atrophy. In order to reverse the atrophy and rebuild the muscle, the area needs to be equally stretched and strengthened on a daily basis. Strengthening alone will leave the muscle tight and unbalanced, making it susceptible to future injury.

Do a full-body ESSENTRICS workout (30 minutes every day) to keep your body balanced with equal strength and range of motion, along with any strengthening that your therapist advises. You will be like new in no time.

Step 3: Once the muscles are strong, return to a normal training schedule

After strengthening the injured muscles, get back to business and continue a regular fitness routine for the rest of your life. Without regular exercise, injuries and pain may return and the body will age more rapidly. ESSENTRICS is an ideal program for maintaining a strong flexible body that heals quickly and is resistant to injury.

HEALING SPECIFIC CONDITIONS

Most injuries and chronic pain are caused by compressed and unbalanced joints. Conditions in this category include osteoarthritis, frozen shoulder, plantar fasciitis, chronic inflammation of the groin, shin splints, hip and knee degeneration, osteoporosis, and chronic back pain. Unless we correct the cause of the problem and heal the original injury, we will be forced to live in chronic pain, suppressing it with medication, and bandaging over the symptoms with temporary solutions such as heat, ice, and massages. ESSENTRICS is so successful in healing injuries and reducing chronic pain because its primary objective is to simultaneously lengthen and strengthen the muscles; this directly relieves compression and rebalances the muscles surrounding the joint.

The following section gives a brief overview and description of some of the most common medical conditions and injuries that ESSENTRICS has had success in relieving and healing. Some of these conditions cannot be fully reversed but can be prevented from progressing further. Others can be greatly improved and sometimes healed completely. (Note: These descriptions are not to be used for self-diagnosis. If you require a diagnosis for one of these conditions, talk to your doctor.)

Every case is unique and depends on many factors, such as age, previous level of fitness, and weight. Your degree of pain relief and injury healing will be as individual as you are, but I can promise you that ESSENTRICS will help you feel better, now and in the future.

Arthritis

"Arthritis" is sometimes used as a catchall term to describe any condition that results in damage to the joints. Arthritis is the leading cause of disability in people over the age of 55, but many young people have arthritis as well. There are many different forms of arthritis, each having a different cause. Physicians often recommend ESSENTRICS to people suffering from osteoarthritis, because the stretching and strengthening help to relieve pain caused by compression and grinding of the joint head due to damaged cartilage.

While it's unfortunately impossible to actually reverse damaged cartilage, we can take all the compression away from the damaged area, thereby totally relieving pain. We can also prevent further grinding and damage of the cartilage.

Forms of arthritis include:

- osteoarthritis, a degenerative joint disease

- rheumatoid arthritis and psoriatic arthritis, autoimmune diseases in which the body is attacking itself

- septic arthritis, which is caused by joint infection

- gouty arthritis, which is caused by uric acid crystals in the joint that cause inflammation

Osteoarthritis, the most common form, occurs most often following a trauma or an infection of the joint. Because of the initial trauma, the muscles surrounding the joint become compressed as they lose their flexibility, usually owing to atrophy. As the muscles shrink, they tighten, compressing the joint, and thus flattening the synovial membrane and squeezing out the synovial fluid. When the joint is compressed, with limited or no lubrication, movement is painful and difficult as the bones rub together (acting like sandpaper) and cause degenerative damage to the joint. That damage and pain in the cartilage are known as osteoarthritis.

As with all joint compression, in order to prevent further damage and relieve the pain, the joints need to be pulled apart, or decompressed, enabling the synovial fluid to enter into the synovial membrane (synovial sack). To prevent further damage, the muscles are strengthened in a lengthened position, decompressing the joint and permitting the synovial fluid to reenter.

Passive stretching and massages are useless for permanent pain relief in arthritic joints. They offer initial relief when a joint is pulled apart, but the moment the person stands up and puts his or her full weight on the joint, the pain will return. The muscles must be strengthened in the lengthened position to be able to prop up the muscles surrounding the joint and keep the joint decompressed. They were created to give that support, and that's what they were like before they atrophied. The lengthening and strengthening required to relieve osteoarthritis are the basic technique used in every ESSENTRICS workout.

Osteoporosis

Bone is the hardest material in the body, except for the nonliving enamel of the teeth. Bone is made up of complex crystalline calcium (with magnesium) salts, which give it the necessary hardness, and is interspersed with strong fibrous strands creating a living matrix. The design of this matrix gives resilience and some elasticity to the hard calcium component.

Bone is a living tissue; cells (called osteocytes) maintain its functional integrity. Bones also have a rich blood supply and bleed when injured, like any other living tissue. Your bones react to exercise in much the same way as your muscles. Exercise leads to increased bone strength; lack of exercise leads to bone weakness. Exercise is the means by which calcium is delivered into the bones. A withdrawal of calcium from the bone leads to loss of density, known as osteoporosis. Fit people can safely subject their bones to stresses and strains in the course of life's many activities, but for someone suffering from osteoporosis the same stresses could lead to fractures.

Bones tend to become weaker with age, particularly in women going through menopause who experience a reduction in the sex hormone estrogen. (But while women are four times more likely than men to develop the condition, men can also have osteoporosis.) We also see osteoporosis far too often in young women who suffer from eating disorders such as bulimia and anorexia. In spite of their light body weight, their bones suffer from a loss of fibrous strands in the living matrix, and this loss causes the bones to become brittle and vulnerable to stress and other fractures.

Osteoporosis is a debilitating condition that can be prevented and, in many cases, reversed. Any bone can be affected, but the most common fractures are in the hip and spine. A hip fracture almost always requires hospitalization and major surgery. It can impair a person's ability to walk unassisted and may cause prolonged or permanent disability.

Regular weight-bearing exercises and a diet rich in calcium are necessary to keep the bones healthy and strong. Many prescription drugs also help reverse osteoporosis (weight-bearing exercise should accompany medication!). But contrary to what most people think, weight-bearing exercises do not require lifting weights. "Weight-bearing exercise" simply means that you put sufficient stress on the full skeleton to gently stress the bones on a daily basis. And the human body is a substantial weight all by itself.

Weight-bearing exercises require you to bend your spine forward, backward, sideways, and rotationally to stress the bones of your torso. We have to stress every one of our 200 bones, not just the most obvious, big ones. We need to bend and straighten our fingers and our feet; we need to lift, lower, bend, and straighten our arms and legs. Lots and lots of big, full-body movements as well as tiny movements are needed to stress the full body's bones!

In addition to stressing the bones, we need to get calcium crystals into them. The combined requirements of stressing the bones and delivering the calcium minerals into them can be met most easily and effectively with large full-body movements, which create a pumping action that enhances the circulation of blood into the bones. And in case you think your morning calcium pill has you covered, know that being sedentary and taking a calcium supplement is not nearly as effective as taking that same supplement and maximizing it with some exercise.

Hip Pain

Because of the amount of force required to walk or jump, the hip joint is required to support many times the weight of the body. This makes hip health very important and hip pain very serious for a person's overall well-being.

The hip joint attaches the leg to the torso. The head of the thighbone (femur) swivels in a socket made up of pelvic bones, called the acetabulum. While many causes of hip pain can arise from the joint itself, there are other parts surrounding the hip that can also be the source of pain. An imbalance in the muscles that attach the leg to the torso can also be the cause of hip pain. Overuse of the hip joint in high-impact activities can lead to compression-related damage of the joint. There are many specific sources of hip pain, including arthritis, injuries to the IT band, fractures, sprains, sciatica, and overuse injuries.

The hip muscles, bursas, and ligaments are designed to shield the joint from the forces it must withstand. When these structures are inflamed, the hip cannot function and pain will occur.

Gentle full-body stretches are generally the fastest way to relieve hip pain like sciatica because they loosen up the contracted muscles that are causing the tension and squeezing of the nerve. Doing nothing—unless so advised by a doctor or physiotherapist—will lead to more shrinkage, atrophy, and increased pain.

Knee Pain

The knee joint joins the thigh with the lower leg, and it's actually two joints—one between the femur and the tibia, and one between the femur and the patella. The knee supports the whole weight of the body and is the joint most vulnerable both to injury and to the development of osteoarthritis.

Injury can happen to any of the ligaments, bursas, or tendons surrounding the knee joint. Injury can also happen to the ligaments, cartilage, menisci (plural of meniscus), and bones forming the joint. The complexity of the design of the knee and the fact that it is an active, weight-bearing joint are factors in making it one of the most commonly injured joints and very prone to pain.

The causes of knee pain include fractures, tendinitis, meniscus tears, ligament tears, cartilage damage (often caused by a sedentary lifestyle), and injury to the ACL (anterior cruciate ligament), a common sports-related injury.

JOINT REPLACEMENT

Over the past few decades, joint replacements have become as commonplace as having a cavity filled. We can avoid these dangerous and costly procedures if we protect the joints from damage in the first place. It's time to learn from the past and focus on prevention by examining what we as a culture are doing to create such a high demand for hip and knee replacements as we grow older.

There are three main reasons for joint replacements: overweight, underused muscles, and overused muscles.

1. Overweight causes trauma to joints: The human body is simply not designed to handle obesity. The joints were not designed to bear excess weight, so overweight causes compression from trauma and joint damage. Eventually the joints wear out and need replacing.

2. Underused muscles compress joints: In every group of muscles in the body, including the knees and hips, underused muscles cause compression from atrophy and joint damage. Eventually the joints wear out and need replacing.

3. Overused muscles compress and cause trauma to joints. Overused muscles are often found in athletes who excessively strengthen the muscles surrounding the joints while both engaging in and training for a sport. The repetitive strength training and constant impact trauma from the sport compress the joints, and the compression leads to joint damage. Overused joints are also found in people who walk heavily, pounding or slamming the ground with each step. Any repetitive abuse will lead to joint damage. If the abuse doesn't stop, eventually the joints wear out and need replacing.

Back Pain

Back pain strikes 80 to 90 percent of the North American population at some time in their lives. Back pain costs the economy billions of dollars in time off work and costs consumers billions in medical bills, medication, visits to therapists, and other treatments.

Although there are many medical causes of back pain, the most common cause is mechanical—unbalanced muscles. As we age, the jellylike substance within the disks of the spinal column slowly dries out and shrinks. When a disk shrinks unevenly, one side of it dries out faster than the other and it takes on a wedge or pie shape. The uneven shrinkage may be due to many things: leaning to one side more than the other, carrying a heavy bag on the same shoulder, carrying a child on the same hip, or throwing or catching a ball with the same arm. Whatever the cause, whenever the disk is lower on one side than the other, the result is the same chain of events. As the spinal muscles try to keep the spine straight, one side has to work to pull the dropped side up, leading to an overworking (and resulting imbalance) of those muscles.

When the overworked muscles become exhausted, they freeze, creating a splint. This involuntary spasm is excruciatingly painful. The surrounding muscles all participate in protecting the exhausted muscle until the back muscles have gone into a rock-hard state of full spasm. When this happens, you may endure an average of 10 days before the muscles release this painful contraction. Anyone who has ever experienced this will attest to the pain and would be willing to do anything rather than experience it twice.

A spasm is the body's way of protecting itself by inhibiting any movement of the exhausted muscles; in effect, a spasm gives the exhausted muscles a rest. Ironically, the body's means of protecting itself is also the source of excruciating pain. The process of disks drying out can begin in our mid-twenties, and ends in our mid-sixties; this is why back pain strikes 25- to 65-year-olds most often.

A full-blown spasm can sometimes last for up to 14 days. After the spasm has been released, we need to focus on preventing a future attack. In order to do this (assuming that the attack was one of the 80 percent caused by unbalanced muscles), we need to keep our muscles permanently balanced. When muscles are balanced, one muscle group will no longer be overloaded. Since 80 percent of back pain is caused by biomechanical imbalance of the muscular skeleton, there is an 80 percent likelihood (statistically) that someone suffering from back pain has unbalanced muscles.

ESSENTRICS was developed partially to relieve back pain. Many sufferers claim that after doing the program, they stopped having acute bouts of back pain. Many people have claimed to be "cured," but back pain is not a disease—it is a condition. You don't cure it; you control it. Control can feel like a "cure," but if you stop exercising, the back pain will most likely return.

If the cause of the pain was an uneven disk, that problem won't go away until the disk dries out completely and becomes even again. Anyone who has ever tried them knows that—just as with most injuries—regular stretching and strengthening exercises are the easiest and fastest way to get rid of back pain.

You've learned so much about *what* ESSENTRICS does for the body; now it's time to learn *how* to do it. In Part III, you can choose from several different workouts, each designed to help you with specific conditions, and each one guaranteed to help wake up your mitochondria, ignite your metabolism, prevent chronic diseases, generate new brain cells, give you more energy, and help you develop a long, lean, dancer's body—all in 30 minutes a day. Let's get started!

PART III

THE EIGHT AGE-REVERSING WORKOUTS

CHAPTER 9

HOW TO DO THE WORKOUTS

Many of us want to look 10 years lighter and 10 years younger than we do today. We need good posture and strong and flexible muscles to succeed. We want to reverse any atrophy that might be making us feel weak or inflexible or less energetic. The first thing we have to do is to reverse the atrophy with a series of flexibility and strengthening exercises.

I'm excited to share these workouts with you, because I have seen such amazing results in everyone who has ever committed to doing ESSENTRICS for 30 minutes a day. You've seen the research: You know that the eccentric approach to exercise is the safest, most efficient, and most powerful means of stretching and strengthening. You know that your body will become more balanced and flexible, and you'll remain injury-free. You know you can develop the "dancer's body" you've always wanted, with longer, leaner muscles and a much higher concentration of energy-producing, fat-burning mitochondria powering your cells. You'll wake up every muscle in your body, reverse the aging process, tell your DNA you're alive and you need every single cell in your body—no premature cell loss for you! You are ready to *Age Backwards*.

When starting these exercises, take your time and don't overexert yourself. For the first week or two, do your 30 minutes a day but make sure you are moving gently and relaxing while doing the exercises. Actually, you will strengthen faster if you *don't* try to strengthen the muscles. Staying relaxed will get you a lot further than overpushing yourself and getting discouraged and quitting!

If you are in great shape, you may wonder if these exercises could possibly strengthen you. Remember the story of Anik, the injured ballet dancer who came back even stronger after two weeks of doing ESSENTRICS? Try it! The results will speak for themselves.

If you are out of shape or weak or suffering from any degree of atrophy, any exercises will be more difficult. But please don't get discouraged. Your arms will feel as if they weigh a ton. You might find that just straightening your back even a small amount will make you sweat profusely, and shake. Keep trying 20 to 30 minutes a day, not more. From my experience, within 2 weeks these exercises will suddenly become easier and you won't sweat anymore.

I am always so impressed by how resilient the human body is; how ready it is to be revitalized when given half a chance, no matter how bad a shape we might be in.

BE A SMART EXERCISER

These ESSENTRICS workouts are designed to be done every day for approximately half an hour. The human body responds well to half an hour of daily exercise that does not cause injury or make you a fitness fanatic. All you need to stay in shape is 30 minutes of these full-body stretching and strengthening workouts. Doing too much, like doing too little, can create its own series of problems. The important thing is consistency.

If you feel a sharp, "knifelike" pain when doing any exercises, stop immediately. Knifelike pain is a warning that your body is incapable of doing the exercises safely; continuing might lead to injury. However, if you just find them difficult and tiring, keep going; they are supposed to be challenging.

As you try these workouts, take note of how quickly your body responds to the challenges. Marvel at how remarkably receptive the human body is to stimulus, and how it adapts itself quickly and efficiently anytime new demands and stresses are placed upon it. Miraculous! Even if you have never exercised in your life, or have allowed your body to stagnate with inactivity, your muscles will respond rapidly to

TWO RULES TO FOLLOW IN EVERY ESSENTRICS WORKOUT

Rule 1: Use Circular Movements

ESSENTRICS is based on a functional concept of interlocking circles or wheels. We recognize that the body is not flat but three-dimensional and capable of moving in a circular-type motion. This program is designed to reflect the reality of natural circular movement of the body: that the arms perform a circular motion within the sockets, that the torso performs a circular-type motion using the flexibility of the spine, and that the legs perform a circular motion within the hip sockets.

Rule 2: Balance the Body

ESSENTRICS improves your posture and tones your body overall. However, in order for this program to work there is one unbreakable rule; the entire body must be worked out in the same session so as to completely rebalance all muscles and joints. In order for us to achieve the overall long, lean look of ESSENTRICS, every muscle must be equally engaged.

strength and flexibility training, and the benefits of this training will fuel your desire to keep progressing and challenging yourself.

MAKING EXERCISE A HABIT

The best time to exercise? *Anytime you will do it!* Work with your biorhythms to find the time of day when you enjoy exercising the most and are least likely to let it slide. Doing your exercise first thing in the morning will help you build a consistent habit. After all, if you do your workouts before anything else, the rest of your life won't have a chance to get in the way! But if lunchtime is better, or an hour before bed works for you, go with that—just commit to your 30 minutes a day, no matter what. Do it for your cells, your heart, your muscles, your brain! According to a study at the University of Copenhagen, just *one session* of intense exercise will improve your long-term memory.[54] But consistency is essential, and those brain benefits, while impressive, will wear off if you don't keep exercising.

Most important of all, have fun doing these. They will make your body feel so good that you'll feel you can't possibly be exercising. Forget "no pain, no gain"—your body knows what's good for it. Your body will thank you for making it feel so relaxed, so full of energy and oxygen, and so young!

CHAPTER 10

STRAIGHTEN YOUR POSTURE

Good posture gives you the appearance of confidence and youth and it also pulls your spine upward, opening space for all your organs to function comfortably in the space "God" intended for them.

The rounded shoulders and curved spine of poor posture make you look tired and old while reducing the space intended for your organs. The shrinking of the spine pushes the organs downward, making them squish outward because they have nowhere else to go. This makes us look fatter than we actually are! In other words, good posture makes us look younger and slenderer and bad posture makes us look older and fatter! Take your choice.

However, improving your posture and straightening your back can be a daunting task if your muscles are weak or are in any degree of atrophy. When our muscles are strong and flexible, maintaining good posture is easy, natural, and comfortable. And when muscles are strong and flexible, keeping the back straight for extended periods of time is easier and more comfortable than slouching. The spine is designed for a lifetime of good posture, but the only way to keep it that way is to exercise it. Movement is essential to maintaining good posture, particularly if we spend upwards of 8 hours a day sitting at a desk and the rest of our day on a sofa in front of the TV.

If looking great is not motivation enough, consider that good posture is also essential for healthy organ function. Poor posture negatively affects every system in the body—cardiovascular, neurological, digestive, and skeletal.

Poor posture impedes the ability of our lungs to inhale adequate quantities of oxygen, leading to oxygen deprivation in the brain and muscles, and making us feel chronically tired and sluggish. Poor posture also puts pressure on the digestive system that can cause heartburn, gas, cramps, bloating, and constipation. Poor posture prevents the cardiovascular system from achieving good circulation of energy-giving blood.

Poor posture is often the result of a sedentary lifestyle. Inactivity leads directly to atrophy: The hundreds of muscles required to hold the spine upright weaken and the slippery slope of rapid aging begins.

Weak atrophied muscles cannot support the spine in an erect position for longer than a few minutes without becoming exhausted and collapsing. If your muscles are weak, maintaining good posture is grueling, even unattainable. But don't despair; our muscles are waiting and ready for us to strengthen them. All we have to do is a little bit of exercise on a daily basis, and within a few short weeks we should have stunning posture.

The God-given muscles in the body are actually designed to be strong and capable of lasting a lifetime. They are not designed to be weak! A little bit of work and they will strengthen rapidly.

The spine is made up of 33 small, wedge-shaped bones called vertebrae, which form a gentle double-S curve starting at the base of the skull and ending at the tailbone. The shape of the double-S curve gives flexibility to the spine, which resembles an accordion as it compresses and expands. When we pull the spine upward it lengthens and we look taller, and when we allow the spine to compress, we look shorter. We actually would be taller or shorter if we were to be measured at our different postural positions.

The torso has hundreds of muscles at its disposal to help us maintain good posture. These muscles range from small to large and run from the spine to our shoulders, ribs, skull, legs, or hips. They work in concert to keep the spine strong, flexible, and in healthy alignment. Every single one of these muscles plays a vital role in good posture and every one must be strengthened and stretched equally in order for the spine to remain balanced. When our spinal muscles are balanced we have comfortable perfect posture.

The spine is intended to move in every direction imaginable; therefore, we need to do exercises to keep the spinal muscles capable of moving in all directions.

It might seem a daunting challenge to exercise all the muscles that are required to achieve good posture, but I will show you that, in fact, it is quite simple. The only part that is difficult is your personal commitment to your body! Are you ready to do these exercises at least three times a week for the rest of your life?

I have put together a sample of exercises that will give you both strength and flexibility in all the muscles required for good posture. These exercises also have many other benefits, such as helping you control your weight, and toning your torso to give you an attractive shape.

Your mother probably reminded you to "stand up straight!" And she was correct, but sometimes we're not quite sure what "straight" means. Fitness and sports training commonly overstrengthen the shoulder, arm, and upper back muscles in the misguided belief that this will develop good posture. But there is a great difference between a strong, rigid, immobile back and a strong, straight, fully mobile back.

Strengthening must be balanced by an equal degree of dynamic flexibility; otherwise it is dangerous and counterproductive, leading to premature atrophy. Anyone who is engaged in any form of fitness activity or sport should take a step back to examine the results. Ask yourself if your activity causes more problems than it is solving. It is very difficult to admit that the training we have become passionate about could be harming us. It is hard to admit that an instructor whom we respect and who's probably become a friend is giving us workouts that are actually causing us harm. Life is often about choices and facts and even fitness activity that is bad for you becomes difficult to break away from.

That being said about the fitness industry, the absolutely worst thing we can do for our posture is to be sedentary! Being sedentary will inevitably lead to rapid aging, irreversible atrophy, and poor posture. Poor posture puts us on the slippery slope of cardio, digestive, skeletal, and neurological problems.

Life is fun—so we shouldn't let our bodies get in the way of living!

CEILING REACHES

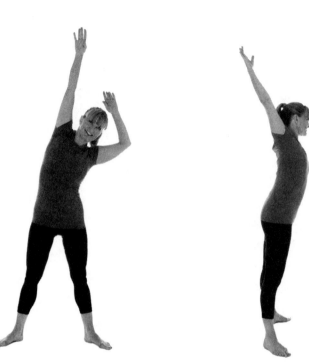

Reach one arm as high as possible, keeping the other arm bent near the head. As you are reaching toward the ceiling, breathe in and out slowly 3 times. With the release of each breath, try to stretch toward the ceiling a little more. You should feel a gentle tug in the rib muscles, the spine, and the abs.

When you cannot reach any higher toward the ceiling, then gently pull the extended arm toward the back. You should feel a tug at the front of your shoulder joint. Hold for one deep breath and then relax the muscles but keep the arm above the head. This backward movement will help straighten the spine and improve posture. Alternate the ceiling reaches 16 times.

HAMSTRING STRETCHES

Lying flat on your back, keeping one knee bent with your foot flat on the ground, lift one leg, holding it wherever you can reach it. It is important to keep your back flat on the ground. Many people need to bend their knee slightly if their hamstring muscles are too tight to keep the leg straight. The objective is to stretch the hamstring muscle, not to straighten the leg. Do 1½ minutes per leg. Repeat twice for each leg, alternating legs between sequences.

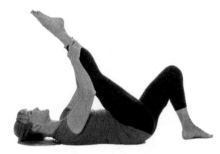

HAMSTRING STRETCH MODIFICATIONS

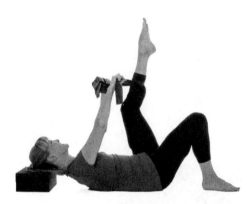

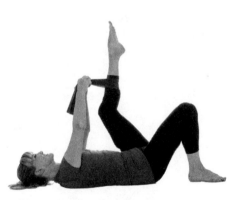

If you have a rounded back and are unable to rest your head comfortably on the floor, use a cushion. You will protect your spine by raising your head and reducing the compression on the cervical spine.

If you can't reach your leg while keeping your back flat on the ground, wrap a theraband around your lower leg to help pull it toward you. Many people bend their knee slightly if their hamstring muscles are too tight to keep the leg straight. The objective is to stretch the hamstring muscle, not to straighten the leg.

IT BAND STRETCH

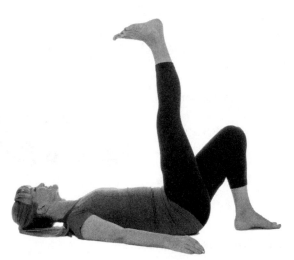

Make sure one knee is bent with the foot flat on the ground in order to protect your spine. Flex the foot of the raised leg. (Note: You should bend the knee of the raised leg if the hamstring is too tight to keep the knee straight.)

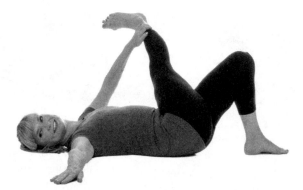

Gently push the extended leg across the body, pushing the leg downward and pulling it toward your chest. When done correctly, this IT band stretch will feel slightly uncomfortable; however, never continue pushing if you feel pain.

BABY STRETCH

Depending on what stretch feels more comfortable for you, you can pick either position 1 or position 2.

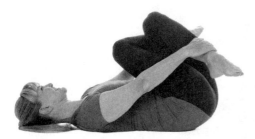

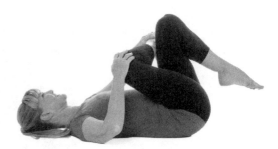

Position 1: Tuck the lower knee under the upper knee while holding both shins with corresponding hands. Slowly swivel your hips side to side in order to feel a stretch in the hip muscles. Keep moving 15 seconds per leg and change legs 4 times.

Position 2: Rest the foot on the opposite knee and pull the thigh toward your chest, keeping your spine flat on the ground. Swivel your hips side to side in order to feel a stretch in the hip muscles.

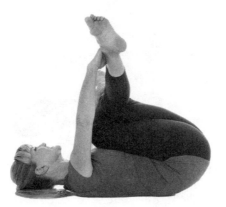

After completing the hip stretches of position 1 or 2, continue into this lower spine stretch. Hold your shins and lift the lower spine slightly off the ground while doing a gentle pelvic tilt. This will increase the flexibility of the vertebrae of your lower spine with the benefits of improving your posture. Slowly swivel your hips side to side to move the spine and unlock tight vertebrae.

PRETZEL EXERCISE

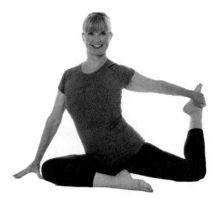

Step 1: Sit with the front leg bent while holding the ankle of the back leg.

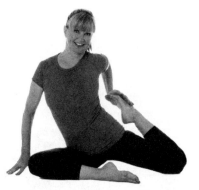

Step 2: Pull heel gently toward the bum. Make sure that the weight of the body is never on the kneecap, but on the thigh. Release the stretch and repeat 3 times slowly, taking 16 seconds per leg.

OPEN CHEST SWAN SEQUENCE FOR POSTURE

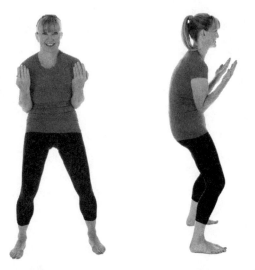

Step 1: Bend your knees and round your back by tucking your tailbone under while slightly bending forward. At the same time bend your elbows, keeping them close to your body with the hands in front of your body.

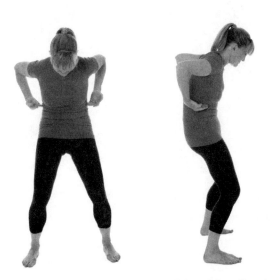

Step 2: Pull the elbows behind you while raising the shoulders.

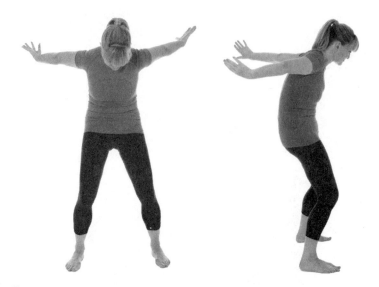

Step 3: Keep the spine rounded and the shoulders raised while straightening the elbows behind you. Simultaneously twist the arms in the shoulder sockets.

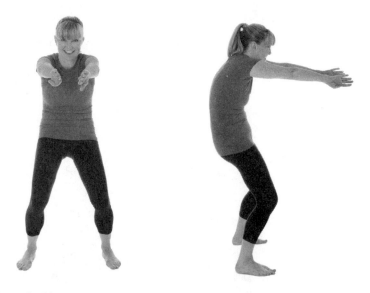

Step 4: Slowly and with resistance sweep the arms to meet in front, keeping the shoulders raised and the arms twisted in the sockets.

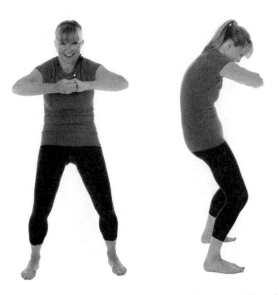

Step 5: Interlock your fingers and draw the hands toward the chest, making sure that your elbows and shoulders remain raised. When your hands are close to your chest try to pull the hands apart but don't release the grip on your fingers. This will give you a lovely stretch between the shoulder blades.

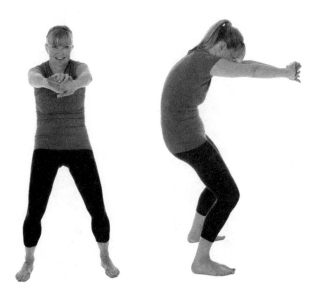

Step 6: Keeping the shoulders raised, slowly straighten the elbows, imagining that you are pushing something forward.

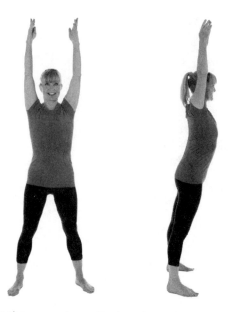

Step 7: Slowly raise the arms above the head, reaching as high as you can toward the ceiling. Be careful not to sink your weight into the lower spine. Keep as straight as possible with your weight always slightly forward.

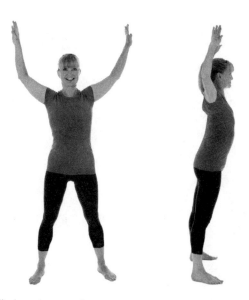

Step 8: Carefully bend your elbows, pointing them toward the back of the room. This movement will stretch the chest muscles.

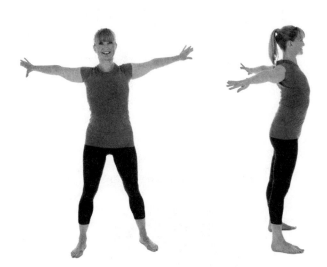

Step 9: Straighten the elbows, keeping the chest open. This will help to stretch and strengthen the entire spine. Repeat steps 1 through 9 three times. Take about 30 seconds to do this entire sequence.

SIDE-TO-SIDE BENDS WITH LUNGE

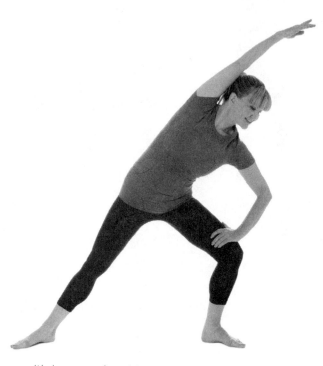

Lunge sideways with legs comfortably apart, making sure that the bent knee is aligned over the arch of the foot. Raise the working arm to be aligned with your ear, keeping the elbow straight. Reach as far away from your body as possible, trying to pull the arm out of the socket (don't worry—it is impossible to do it!). The more you pull the arm, the greater the stretching and toning of the waist and spine muscles. Take 3 seconds per side bend, alternating sides 16 to 32 times.

COMMON MISTAKES IN SIDE LUNGES

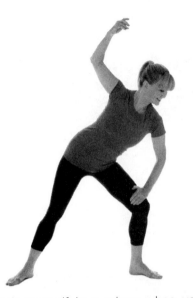

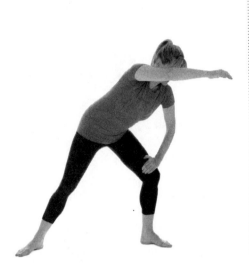

Check yourself in a mirror when you do a side lunge, to be sure you are not making any of these common mistakes. Do not lift the hip of the straight leg and do not let the raised elbow bend—otherwise you will lose the strengthening and flexibility benefits.

Another very common mistake in a side lunge is to let the arm drop in front of the face instead of keeping it next to the ear and head. Make sure you do not rotate the torso toward the floor instead of remaining sideways. These incorrect positions would nullify the waist toning benefits.

SIDE LEG LIFTS

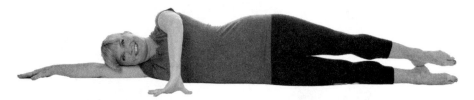

Lie down straight on your side, supporting the upper body with one arm underneath the head and the other hand placed in front.

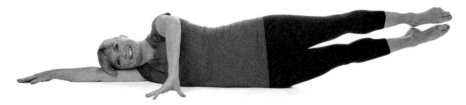

Lift legs upward simultaneously, keeping abs and legs tight. Focus on lengthening the upper and lower body away from each other.

SIT-UPS SEQUENCE FOR POSTURE

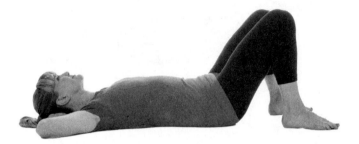

To start a sequence of sit-ups, bend the knees with feet on the floor, lie on your back, place your hands behind your head, and keep the elbows open.

MODIFICATION FOR SIT-UPS

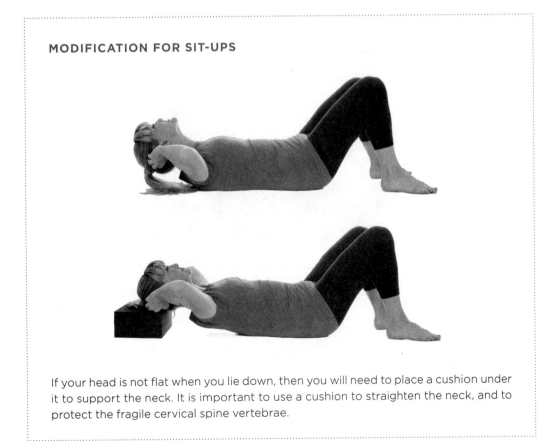

If your head is not flat when you lie down, then you will need to place a cushion under it to support the neck. It is important to use a cushion to straighten the neck, and to protect the fragile cervical spine vertebrae.

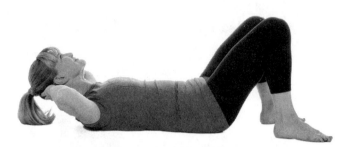

Step 1: Begin the sit-up by lifting the shoulders off the floor. Keep the elbow open throughout the exercise. Then slowly lower the head to the ground. For each sit-up, you should take 3 seconds to lift the shoulders and 3 seconds to lower them. Repeat 16 to 32 times.

Tip: Make sure you keep your neck in line with your spine and keep the abdominal muscles engaged.

COMMON MISTAKES IN SIT-UPS

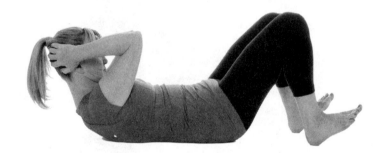

Notice in this photo that the elbows and the head are pulling the body forward. Not only does this forceful use of the neck cause neck pain; it is also dangerous for the spine. Equally important is that it does not use the abdominal muscles, and so no strengthening or toning is achieved.

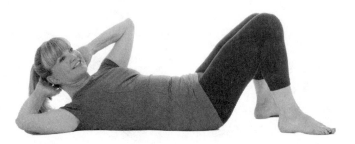

Step 2: Rotate the upper body to do oblique sit-ups, which will strengthen the rib muscles and tone the waist. Keep both hands under the head and repeat 8 times on one side before changing sides.

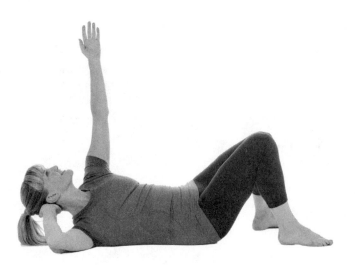

Step 3: Try to touch the ceiling with your fingers as you do the oblique sit-up. These sit-ups will lengthen the waist and abdominal muscles as you strengthen them, helping develop good posture and a strong flexible torso. Repeat 8 on one side before changing sides.

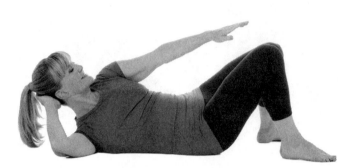

Step 4: Try reaching to the opposite knee as you do these oblique sit-ups. These will strengthen the obliques and abdominal muscles. Repeat 8 on one side before changing sides.

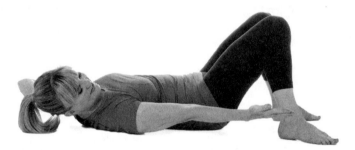

Step 5: Try to touch your heel as you do these oblique sit-ups. These sit-ups will strengthen the waist and spine, helping develop good posture and a strong flexible spine. Repeat 8 on one side before changing sides.

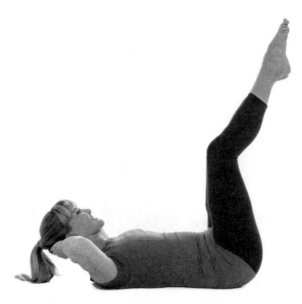

Step 6: Lift both legs as high as possible, keeping the knees bent. Repeat 8 simple sit-ups of the torso.

Note: If you have a weak back always keep one foot on the floor to protect the spine. This is a rule that you should follow whenever exercises require two legs off the floor; you should automatically keep one leg on the floor.

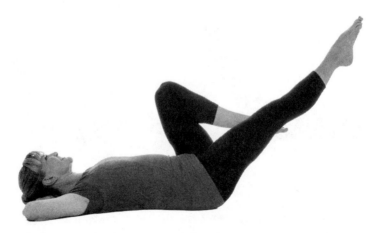

Step 7: Making sure that you press the lower ab muscles into the floor, simultaneously push the straight leg downward, using strong resistance. Repeat 16 to 32 slow-motion bicycles.

RESISTANCE LEG LIFTS (ADVANCED)

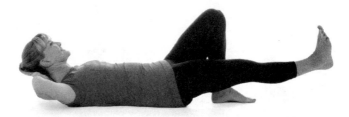

Place your hands behind your head, straighten one leg, and flex the foot. Do a crunch while simultaneously lifting the straight leg off the floor. Do not bring the leg higher than you see it in the image. Press your lower abs into the floor throughout the exercise. Repeat 8 times, then switch legs.

ADVANCED SIT-UPS

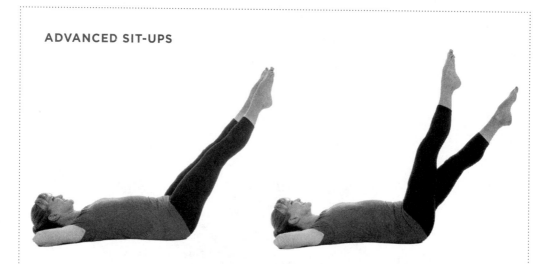

Keep your back flat on the ground and use only the abdominal muscles in this advanced sit-up sequence. (If you are a beginner, do not do these sit-ups.) Extend your legs at a 45-degree angle to the floor. Do 16 fast mini scissors and return to both feet flat on the floor with your knees bent in order to release the strain on your spine between sequences. Repeat scissors 2 to 4 times.

SPINE ROTATIONS

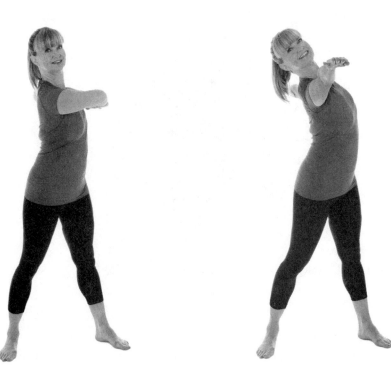

Rotate on spine to one side with arms folded in toward chest, keeping them parallel to the ground. This exercise is to increase the mobility of your spine and improve your posture. Rotate carefully, easing into the stretch. Never force a stretch.

Extending one arm in front and the other behind will help deepen the stretch of the spine. Alternate spine rotations, moving constantly, counting 6 seconds per rotation. Do 8 to 16 spine rotations.

ZOMBIE

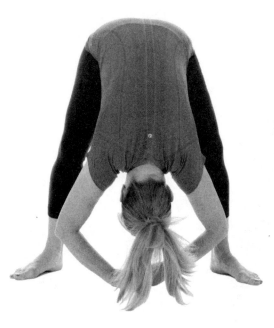

Completely relax the upper body, bending forward with knees bent and arms relaxed. Sway slowly side to side, 4 seconds per side, a minimum of 8 times. Slowly straighten your back to stand straight, rolling up one vertebra at a time.

CHAPTER 11

SPEED YOUR WEIGHT LOSS

As we've discussed throughout the book, if we don't exercise enough, we lose an average of 7 to 8 percent of our cells a decade. If we are sedentary, this cell loss is exacerbated by atrophy. With every muscle cell lost, we also lose thousands of mitochondria, the organelles that are found by the thousands in muscle cells and are responsible for burning a significant amount of the body's calories.

The loss of mitochondria makes it more difficult to burn the calories we consume each day. This effect leads to difficulty controlling our weight, and ultimately to weight gain. Those unspent calories have to go somewhere and so the body converts them into fat to be stored for later use. The main fat storage units are in the hips and stomach, and in and around certain other organs. As our muscles shrink, our insulin sensitivity wanes and we develop a diabetic-like shape—we get skinny legs and arms and expanded fat in the stomach, the hips, and some organs—the opposite of what we want! This muscle loss is the major underlying cause of changes in body shape associated with aging, and it is entirely preventable!

Two aspects of fitness can help us manage our weight:

1. A full-body workout of 30 minutes every day to prevent any of our 620 muscles from atrophying.

2. Using our largest muscles to burn as many calories as possible during that workout.

The trigger for burning calories is muscle activation, and our largest muscles are found between the waist and knees. I refer to these as the "weight loss" group of muscles: the abdominals, gluteus muscles, quadriceps, and hamstrings. We need to engage them to tap into their fat-burning potential.

For those who despise cardiovascular workouts such as running on a treadmill (I'm one of those people), I have put together a series of exercises that I do to prevent my muscles from shrinking and atrophying while burning the maximum possible number of calories. I do these particular exercises two to three times a week to keep the furnaces of my muscle cells stoked! I will do extra pliés throughout the day, just for the fun of knowing that each time I do them, I am burning off extra calories and waking up my mitochondria, giving myself more energy and more calorie-burning power for next time.

LEG LIFT SEQUENCE

Do all the exercises on one leg, then turn over and do them on the other leg. Take 3 minutes to do the full sequence on each leg, for a total of 6 minutes. Note: The hips should always be stacked one on top of the other.

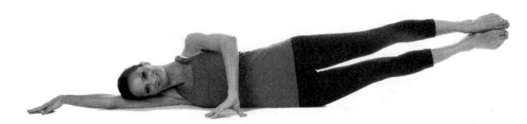

Step 1: Lie down on one side of your body with both legs straight and place the upper arm in front to stabilize the torso. Raise the legs as high as possible (as shown in photo) and return them to the floor. Make sure that you do not use your torso: Use only the legs. Do 8 to 16 leg lifts.

Tip: Imagine that your inner thighs are glued together as you do the exercise.

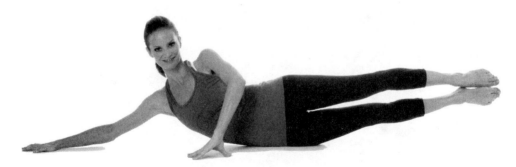

Step 2: Add a sit-up along with the leg lifts. Lift the upper body as you lift the legs, then lower the body as you lower the legs to the floor. Do 8 to 16 per side.

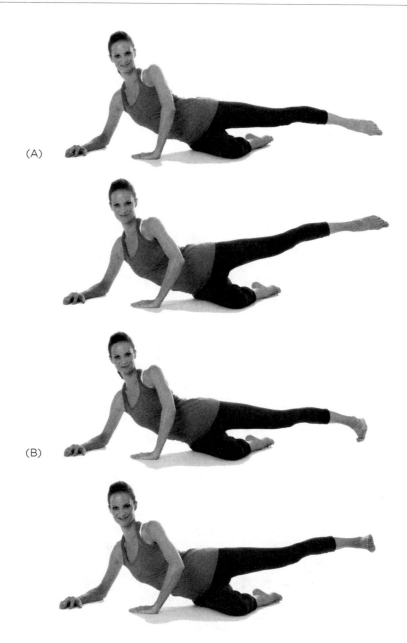

(A)

(B)

Step 3: Lift the body and support the position with your elbow: Bend the lower leg, bringing the knee toward the front while supporting the upper body on the elbow (A). Make sure the side of the leg (the saddlebag area) is facing upward. Pull the upper leg away from the hips (B). This constant pulling out of the hips will decompress them while making the calories burn. Pump the leg up and down 8 to 16 times with your toes alternately pointed and flexed. The leg should not lift very high but should always remain off the floor.

(A)

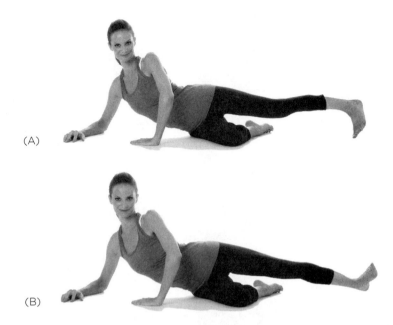

(B)

Step 4: Continue pulling the leg away from the body with a flexed foot. Internally rotate the leg so that the heel points upward (A), then externally rotate the leg so that the heel points down (B). Rotating the leg within the hip socket will improve mobility in the hips. Do 8 full rotations.

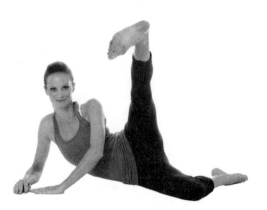

Step 5: Extend the leg in front of the body and slowly lift and lower the leg 8 times.

Modification: If you have a weak or injured back, always keep the knee slightly bent to relieve the load that a straight knee would put on the spine.

PLIÉS SEQUENCE

This plié sequence takes roughly 3 minutes to complete and burns a tremendous number of calories.

To protect the knees, keep them in line with the ankles. If you want to increase difficulty, bend into a deeper plié. Never hold a plié move. The constant movement will keep the muscles thin and flexible while increasing strength.

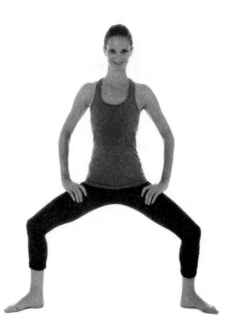

To prepare for a plié, place the legs in a wide stance with feet slightly turned out. Imagine you are against a wall in order to keep your back straight.

Modification: If you have tight hips, you may need to lean slightly forward to maintain balance.

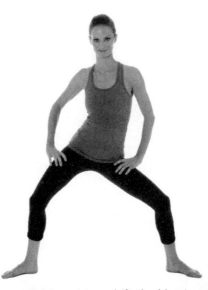

Step 1: Maintaining the basic plié position, shift the hips to one side, return to the center, then shift to the other side. As you shift the hips, immobilize the upper body to ensure that movements happen below the waist. Take your time in each position to get maximum flexibility of the lower spine. Shift the hips 8 times.

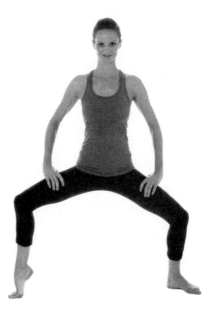

Step 2: Maintaining a basic plié position, lift one heel off the floor, then imagine you are squeezing an orange under your heel as you bring it down. Lifting the heel as high as you can will improve flexibility in the feet. Repeat heel raisers 4 times with each foot.

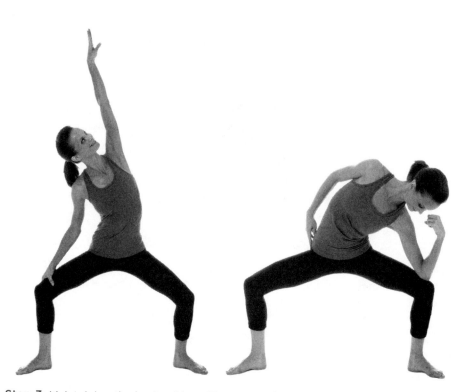

(A)

(B)

Step 3: Maintaining the basic plié position, extend one arm to the ceiling, reaching as far up as possible (A). Imagine you are grabbing a rope from the ceiling, then pull the elbow toward the knee, crunching at the waist (B). Repeat movement 8 times on each side.

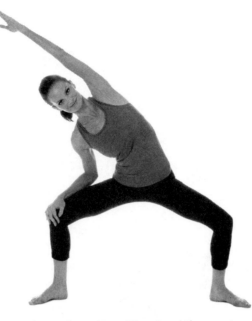

Step 4: Keeping the knees bent in a plié, extend the arm to one side as far as possible. This will tone the waist and improve posture. Alternate sides 16 times.

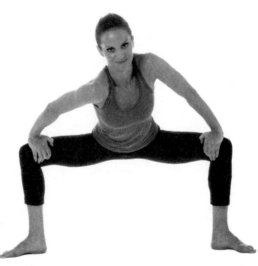

Step 5: Maintaining the basic plié position, place hands on the thighs and try to press the legs open. This will improve flexibility in the hips.

PULLING WEEDS SEQUENCE

Repeat for 3 sequences on each side, for a total of 3 minutes.

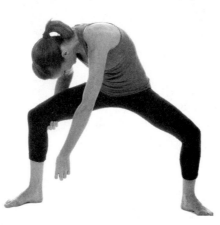

Step 1: Start the sequence by keeping feet in a wide stance, bending the knees, and leaning forward with a rounded back.

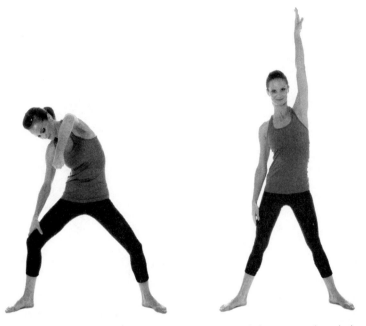

Step 2: Imagine that you are pulling a weed out of the ground and slowly roll up the spine into a standing position with the arm pulling up to the ceiling. The full movement should take 6 to 10 seconds.

Tip: Create resistance in the arm by contracting your muscles throughout the movement.

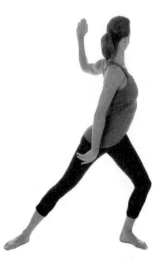

Step 3: Once the arm reaches toward the ceiling, slowly rotate on the spine and push the arm behind you. At the same time, bend the knee into a lunge. This sequence will relieve tight back muscles and improve flexibility in the spine. Take 6 seconds to rotate the spine. Repeat 3 "pulling weeds" sequences on each side.

SIDE BENDS

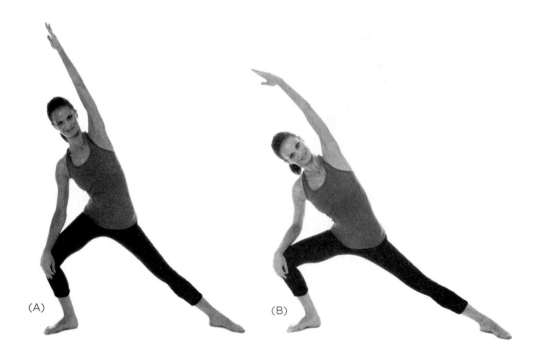

(A)   (B)

Place the legs in a wide stance with feet slightly turned out. Raise the arm next to the ear, keeping it straight while pulling the arm away from the shoulder as much as possible (A). In a side lunge position bend the torso sideways, pulling the top arm until you feel a deep stretch in the ribs (B). Make sure that the hip stays down in order to maintain the side stretch. This will strengthen the core and thin the waist while burning calories.

Alternate sides 8 to 16 times, moving under your muscles' control and not using momentum to throw the body.

Tip: Make sure the arm stays beside the head in order to target the waist and side muscles.

DIAGONAL REACHES

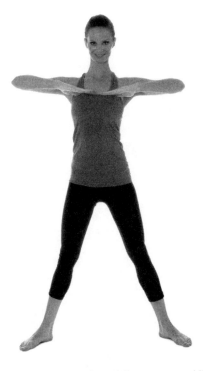

Step 1: Place the feet in a wide stance, bend the arms, and lift the elbows to shoulder height. This position is used as the transition between diagonal reaches as you alternate sides to center and protect the spine.

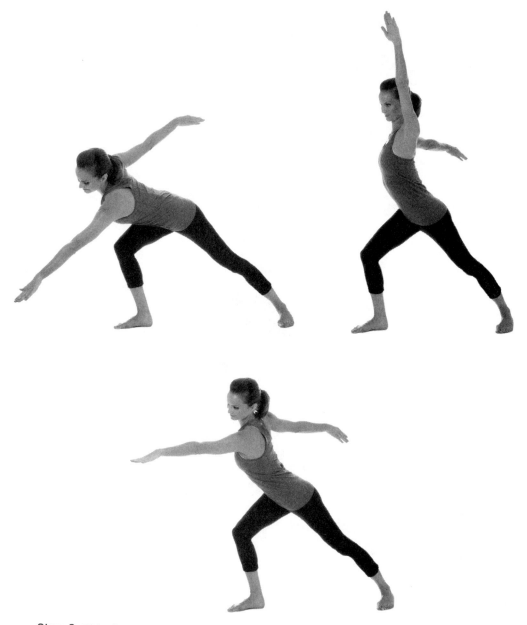

Step 2: This diagonal front lunge alternates sides at three different heights: floor, shoulder, and ceiling. Reach the front arm on a diagonal, pulling the opposite arm behind you. Alternating sides, diagonally lunge at all three heights, passing through the preparation position each time. Do between 8 and 16 diagonal lunges.

Diagonal lunges will increase the flexibility and strength of your spine while improving your posture.

SIT-UPS SEQUENCE

To start a sequence of sit-ups, bend the knees with feet on the floor, lie on your back, place your hands behind your head, and keep the elbows open.

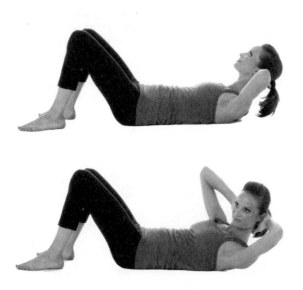

Step 1: Begin the sit-up by lifting the shoulders off the floor. Keep the elbows open and your head off the floor, rotate the shoulders from one side to the other, then lower the head slowly to the ground.

Tip: Make sure you keep your neck in line with your spine and keep the abdominal muscles engaged. Remember to use a cushion to support the neck, if needed (see page 145).

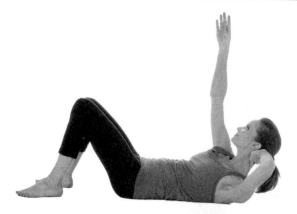

Step 2: Raise one arm to the ceiling and slowly do 8 sit-ups while reaching the arm up. Complete 8 sit-ups with the other arm reaching toward the ceiling.

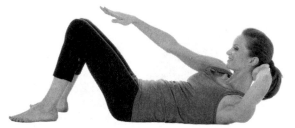

Step 3: Stretch one arm toward the opposite knee and slowly do 8 sit-ups. Repeat 8 times with the other arm.

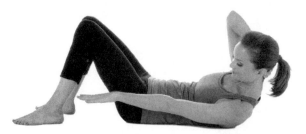

Step 4: Try to touch your ankle by stretching the arm down the side of your body. This exercise will strengthen your obliques. Complete 8 times, then change sides.

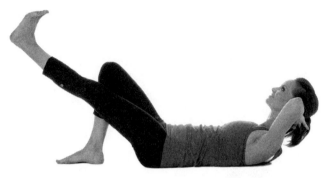

Step 5: Place hands behind the head and straighten one leg with a flexed foot. Do a crunch and simultaneously lift the straight leg off the floor. Do not bring the leg higher than you see it in the image. Repeat 8 times, then switch legs.

ADVANCED SIT-UPS

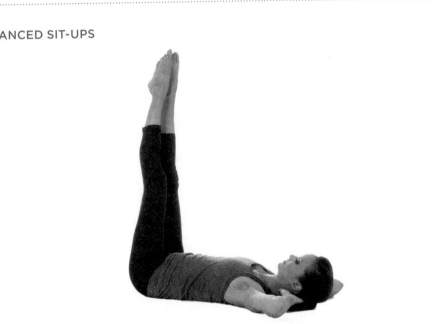

Step 6: Keep your head on the floor and raise both legs in the air. (You may bend your knees if you cannot keep them straight.) Try to lift the pelvis slightly off the floor 8 times. The lifts will target your lower abs.

Tip: Keep the abdominal muscles engaged. If you want extra support, place your arms beside your body. If you have weak back muscles, keep your feet on the floor.

ADVANCED SIT-UPS

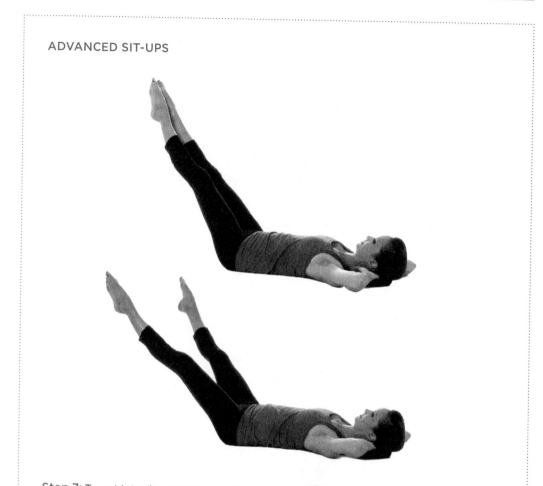

Step 7: To get into the starting position, place the head on the floor with elbows open and lift the legs straight up to the ceiling. Slightly lower your legs toward the floor. Make sure you can keep your abdominal muscles engaged at all times. Open and close legs 8 times.

Tip: If you have a back injury or weak abs, keep the knees slightly bent at all times, and do not bring the legs low to the ground.

ADVANCED SIT-UPS

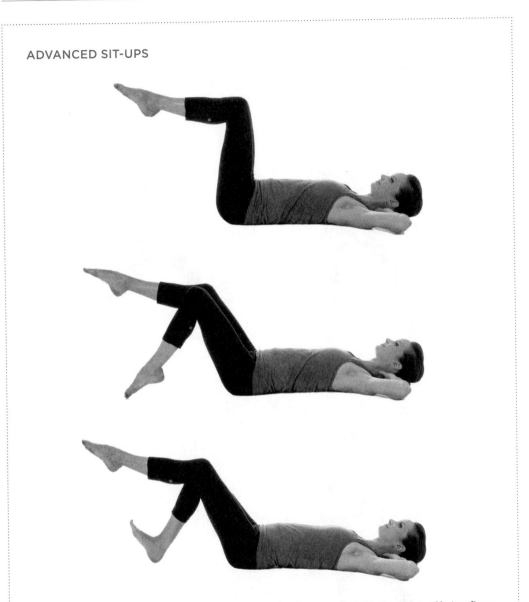

Step 8: Keep the head on the floor, bend the knees, and lift the feet off the floor. In order to be in the starting position, the knees need to be at a 90-degree angle to the chest. Touch one foot on the ground and then bring it back to neutral position. Repeat 8 times, alternating legs. Now repeat the exercise with a flexed foot and gently tap the heel toward the floor. Repeat 8 times, alternating legs.

SQUASH LUNGES

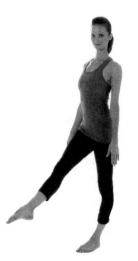

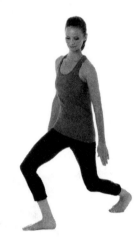

Step 1: Start upright with one leg lifted in front.

Step 2: Carefully drop on the front leg, contracting the muscles around the knee to absorb the impact when you land. Try to land slowly and without making any noise. Bend your back leg.

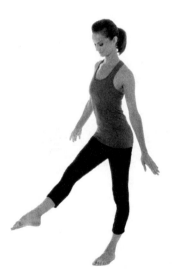

Step 3: Push away from the ground, and return to your original starting position. This sequence of three steps will strengthen the quad and burn calories. Repeat 4 to 8 squash lunges with each leg.

DIAGONAL LEVER STRETCHES

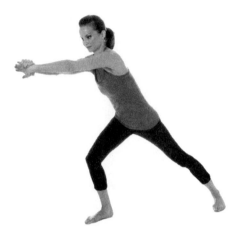

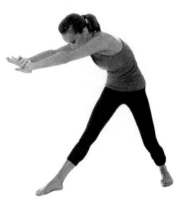

Step 1: In a deep front lunge hold both hands and try to reach as far away as possible from your shoulders. You will feel a deep stretch in the upper back and shoulders.

Step 2: Imagine that you are holding on to something in front and shift the weight into a back lunge. The arms will have remained in front, continuing a deep upper back stretch.

This full-body large sequence will strengthen and stretch your upper back and spine, both improving your posture and burning calories.

CHAPTER 12

SOOTHE YOUR JOINTS

While there are many different causes of joint pain and arthritis, the most common, and the one I have seen most often, is lack of movement and the ensuing atrophy. Gentle, daily exercise can do a great deal to relieve, slow down, and even prevent this type of atrophy, which becomes arthritis. All of the exercises in this chapter are good for young and old to decompress the joints and relieve any joint pain.

As we age, if we do not use our muscles, they will slowly shrink and atrophy. Muscles attach bones together, so when they shrink, they pull the bones closer together, squeezing the joints. This is a slow process, imperceptible to us on a day-to-day basis, but the long-term consequences can be devastating after decades of cumulative wear and tear. We start to notice it when it is manifested as decreased joint mobility, stiffness, and pain. These signs that are happening to our muscles are indications of arthritis to follow. We can stop the arthritis from ever happening simply by correct exercising.

In order to slow down the progression of atrophy, and to reverse the damage, we need to do daily flexibility and strengthening exercises, such as Classical Stretch, ESSENTRICS, or tai chi.

For our purposes in joint compression reversal, we never use weight-training machines. In order to decompress the joints, we need to pull them apart. When we strengthen while we stretch the muscles around the joints, we relieve the pressure on the joints and activate the regenerative processes necessary to reverse arthritis and joint pain.

We need to decompress every joint in our body—in our fingers, shoulders, spine, hips, knees, and feet. Consider this: Each foot alone contains 26 bones, 33 muscles, 31 joints, and over 100 ligaments. The two feet together have over one-quarter of the body's bones (200 bones in total).

Where most joints meet, create opportunities for movement, even the slightest amount. Take off your shoes and regain the maximum amount of movement possible in your feet, toes, and ankles.

HIP STRENGTHENING AND MOBILITY

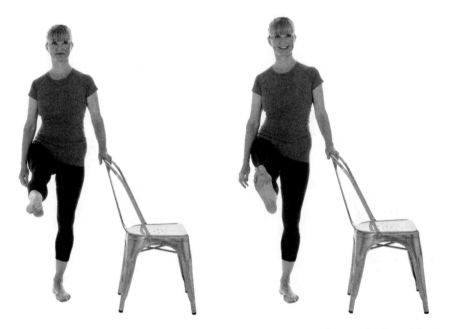

Using a chair, kick the leg in front 8 to 16 times with a pointed foot and a flexed foot. When kicking, try to isolate the leg from the torso by letting only the leg move— not the body. For arthritis relief, height is less important than isolation of the leg and the hip joint.

FOOT, ANKLE, AND KNEE STRENGTHENING

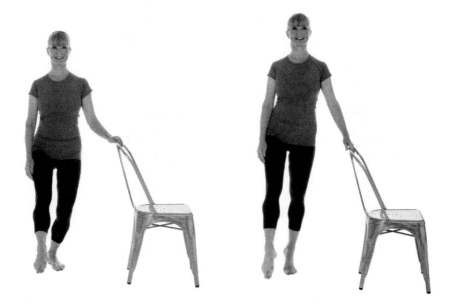

Extend the leg in front while bending the supporting knee (as in a plié). Then straighten the supporting leg and lift the heel. Repeat this sequence slowly 4 times before changing legs. This sequence helps to liberate jammed tight joints, giving them strength and mobility.

HIP STRETCH

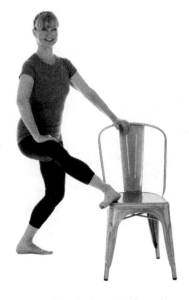

Rest your bent leg on the seat of a chair while keeping your supporting leg bent and your back straight. The exercise will slowly move your hips in as many different directions as possible. Rock your hips backward into an arch, then into a deep tuck underneath, followed by side-to-side swaying of the hips. This will clean out scar tissue in the hip socket, giving greater mobility and ease of hip motion.

SPINE AND HAMSTRING STRETCH

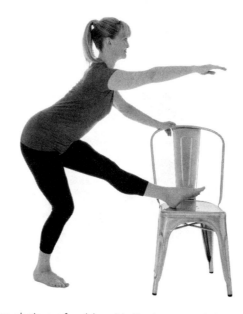

Place your leg on the chair, preferably with the knee straight. Lean forward, keeping your spine as straight as possible while gently extending one arm over the leg. You will feel a tug in the hamstrings and perhaps in your back. Gently move into and out of the stretch; never hold a position, as holding diminishes the flexibility benefits. Keep moving in this hamstring stretch for about 1 minute before changing legs. Repeat this hamstring stretch twice with each leg.

QUAD AND PSOAS STRETCH

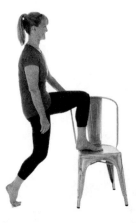

Step 1: Place your foot flat on the seat of the chair. Raise the heel of the standing leg while bending the knee. Do a pelvic tilt as you shift the full weight of the body toward the seat of the chair.

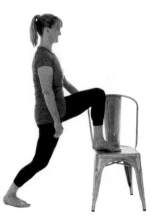

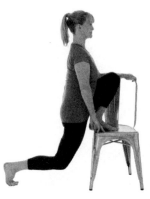

Step 2: Lock your pelvic tilt as you try to replace the heel of the back foot on the floor. You will feel a stretch at the front of your hip. This is stretching a muscle that restricts movement in the lower spine and makes us age rapidly when it is tight. (I call this the "old age muscle"!) This movement should be done slowly: it should take about 15 seconds to complete.

Step 3: Very slowly, lower the knee of the standing leg toward the ground. The moment you cannot lower any farther, slowly straighten up the leg and return to step 1. Repeat steps 1, 2, and 3 on the same leg 3 times very slowly before changing legs. Flexible muscles decompress the tight joints that cause arthritic pain and discomfort.

LONG ADDUCTOR OR INNER THIGH STRETCH

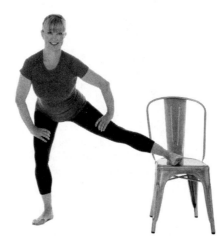

Place your leg comfortably on the seat of the chair. Bend slightly forward while rotating the leg inward. The trick in this stretch is to keep moving the rotation and your forward bend until you find the spot where you feel the inner leg stretch. Gently rock into and out of the stretch for about a minute.

SINGLE ARM CEILING REACH

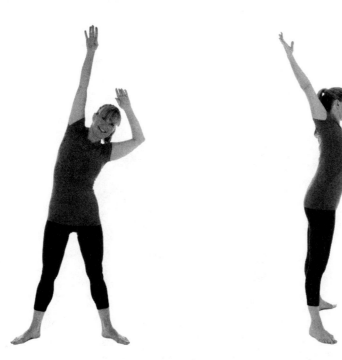

Step 1: Reach one arm as high as possible, relaxing the opposite side of the body. This will allow you to pull the working side of your spine to its maximum degree.

Step 2: Very gently, try to pull the extended arm behind the head as far as is comfortable. This will open the chest and improve posture as well as lengthen the spine and prevent spine arthritis. Take 10 seconds to do steps 1 and 2 before changing arms. Alternate arms at least 4 times.

HOLDING HANDS
IN A FORWARD REACH

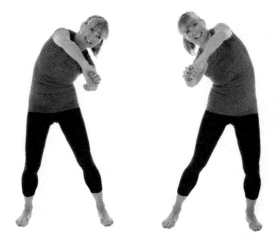

This very popular feel-good stretch works to loosen the spine and upper body. While holding hands in front of you, sway side to side, bending as far sideways as you can to get maximum relief and flexibility. Move very slowly 4 to 8 times side to side, taking the time to really enjoy the feeling of these stretching movements.

FINGERS, WRISTS, AND HANDS

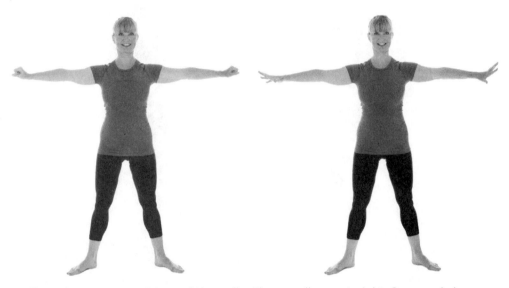

Extend your arms out toward the wall with your elbows straight. Open and close your fists as rapidly as possible. This exercise will strengthen the hands while stretching the muscles of the fingers, helping to prevent and reverse wrist and finger arthritis. Do a minimum of 32 to 64 rapid fist openings and closings.

SHOULDERS, WRISTS, AND HANDS

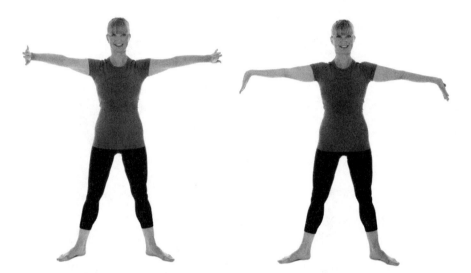

Twist the arms forward and back within the shoulder sockets while keeping the hands flexed and elbows straight. You probably won't like the feeling of this exercise but you will love the results: looser arms and less upper body pain. This sequence increases mobility of the shoulders and spine and reverses atrophy. Repeat 16 slow twists of the arm.

PLIÉS WITH HEEL RAISERS

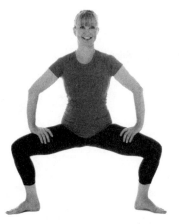 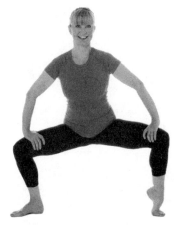

Step 1: Start with feet apart, placing the knees over the mid arch or heels. Keep the stance as wide as you can unless it actually is painful to hold a wide stance. Too wide or too narrow a stance puts undue stress on the knees. Continuously bend and straighten your knees in slow pliés. This movement will strengthen the quads while cleaning scar tissue in the hips. It will also increase the flexibility of your quads, helping to relieve compression on arthritic joints. Do at least 8 slow pliés before adding the heel raisers.

Step 2: Lift one heel only as high as you can. Press the full weight of the body into the lifted heel to stretch the shin as much as possible. Be sure to keep the weight of the foot going through the full five toes. Be sure also not to let the ankle wobble—the ankle must be in clean alignment with the shinbone of the lower leg. Raise and lower the same heel slowly 3 times before changing sides. Repeat both sides twice. Pliés are some of the best exercises to relieve knee, hip, and ankle pain. Try to spend 3 to 4 minutes doing pliés.

Tip: These are the best exercises for knee pain.

SIDE LEG LIFTS

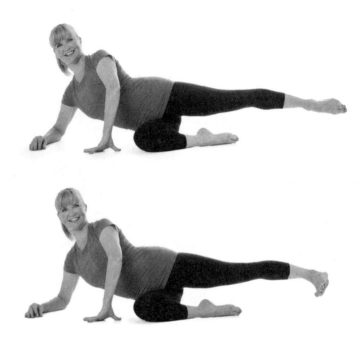

Pull your leg away from your body with the foot pointed. Simultaneously lift your leg as you pull it, taking 3 seconds for each leg lift. Do a minimum of 8 to a maximum of 32 lifts with the foot pointed, as well as 8 to 32 with the foot flexed, before changing to the other leg. These side leg lifts decompress the hip joint, relieving pain and preventing further hip damage.

Tip: These exercises are excellent for hip arthritis.

WASHING TABLES

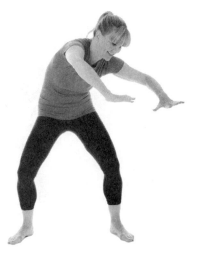

Place your feet apart, your knees and arms bent, and your hands facing downward, fingers spread as though they were going to wipe a tabletop clean with a large cloth. Start bending slightly sideways with a pelvic tilt and your full spine rounded.

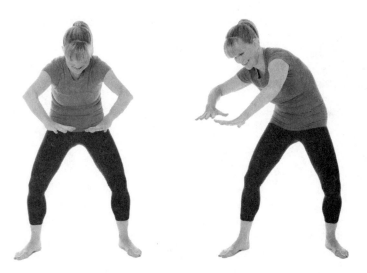

Move from side to side to mimic the action of wiping the top of a very sticky, dirty table. This exercise moves the full spine, upper body, and arms. Do at least 8 wipes of the "table," side to side.

Tip: This movement helps relieve back pain.

WASHING WINDOWS

Start with feet apart, knees and arms bent, and fingers spread out as if to hold a large cloth with which to clean a window. Frame the face with the arms, keeping the elbows well spread apart.

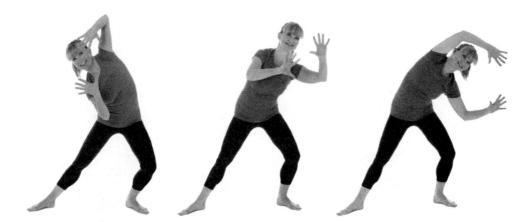

Imagine that you are cleaning a very dirty window and you are sliding your hands across it, but the dirt is sticky and is giving you resistance. Gently shift your weight side to side as you clean the window. Sway gently side to side, washing the window a minimum of 4 to 8 times. This "washing windows" series increases the mobility of your spine, bringing fluids into the vertebrae and reducing back pain.

CHAPTER 13

INCREASE YOUR ENERGY

Even young people can be struck with an energy deficit. If you are working hard, raising kids, trying to keep your head above water, it can be easy to let exercise slide. Please don't! That exercise will give you the power and endurance to get through even the roughest dog-eat-dog days.

As we age, every aspect of our lives tends to slow down. We walk slowly, stand up slowly, get dressed slowly, and even eat slowly. The process of slowing down takes place over a long period of time, making these changes imperceptible to us. The realization that we've slowed down dawns on us most clearly when we are around the young, who generally move at a much faster pace with much less effort.

In some ways slowing down is one of the nicest aspects of aging, because we actually take time to appreciate the world around us. But truth be told, all the middle-aged and older people I know still want to feel like a valuable part of the human race and want to be able to enjoy life. We don't want to give up the option of having a bounce in our step and energy in our bodies. We want to have the choice to move rapidly or slowly! Achieving this requires an understanding of how to maintain energy.

Remember that energy is found in our muscles, in the calorie-burning mitochondria. We need to turn up those furnaces to get energy, and to do that we need to move!

There is a common misconception that to raise your energy levels, you have to run on a treadmill for hours on end. But I've rarely set foot on a treadmill—I've done it less than a dozen times in my life—and I'm full of energy at 65.

One of my jobs is to train Olympic athletes in energy production. When I first start training them I make them compete with me to see who can move fastest. They usually laugh, believing that with their 40-year advantage they'll win, but so far I've always beaten them! That is when they learn to respect the phenomenal power of strong and flexible feet, toes, knees, and hips. Athletes are competitive by nature and so it's easy for me to get them to do foot, ankle, and hip exercises. They all want to beat me and they usually can after a few classes of footwork.

One of my favorite stories about energy is my experience with Joannie Rochette, an Olympic figure skater whose coach had tried every type of training to improve her energy. Athletes often come to me as a last resort, after they have exhausted all other options, and Joannie was no exception. Joannie at 20 years of age didn't have sufficient stamina to finish her long program at full strength and so she was losing valuable points. Her coach thought her lack of energy was due to a weak cardio, so she had her running with professional football players in the hope that this would improve her stamina. But it didn't.

When Joannie arrived at my studio, she was ranked eleventh in the world. After I analyzed her, the first thing I saw was that she had no movement, no mobility, in her toes or ankles. This very common affliction in pro athletes is caused by years of wearing tight skates or running shoes, and never working in bare feet.

Her figure skates prevented any mobility in her ankles or toes, causing premature atrophying of her feet, ankles, calves, and shins. Her atrophy was equivalent to the muscle atrophy seen after someone had been in a cast for weeks. Anyone who has ever been in a cast knows that after a few short weeks the muscles visibly shrink! That's what happened to Joannie's feet. Even though she was only 20, the fact that she had spent her entire life skating meant that her feet had been continually immobilized in skates, and this immobilization had led to weak, skinny muscles and atrophy. The atrophy caused her shins, calves, and feet to become weak and that was the source of her lack of energy.

We spent the next 7 months strengthening and stretching her feet to reverse the atrophy. She proceeded to compete in the Turin Olympics, where she was ranked fifth in the world; and eventually she went on to win a bronze medal at the Vancouver Olympics.

That lesson from Joannie taught me that there are many reasons why we lose our energy, and that it is important not to focus solely on strengthening the cardiovascular system as the only source of energy.

The beauty of strong flexible feet and lower limbs is that they give us not only increased energy but also a bounce in our step. Nothing makes us feel as young and vital as having a spring in our step and energy to spare. Nothing makes us feel as old and worn out as walking a short distance and becoming exhausted.

I have put together a series of exercises that will increase your energy and give you a bounce in your step. I suggest that you do these exercises two to three times a week. You should see a rapid change in your energy and—best of all—you'll feel as though you've turned the clock back 10 years.

BARRE FOOTWORK

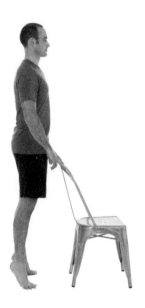

Stand at barre (or sturdy, high-backed chair) with feet apart. Raise and lower heels to work calves. Keep your knees straight. Repeat 8 times.

Bend knees, keeping heels firmly on the ground to target calves.

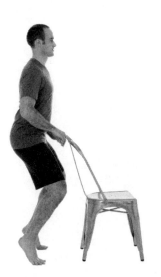

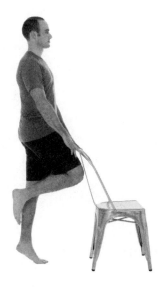

Raise and lower heels with knees bent, using barre or chair for support. Repeat 8 times.

Standing on one leg and, keeping the other leg bent, raise and lower the heel. Repeat 4 times with each foot.

CALF STRETCH SEQUENCE

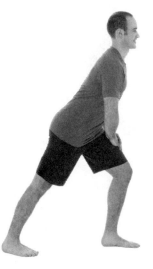 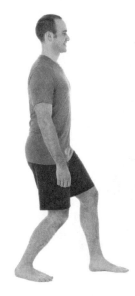

Step 1: Start with one leg extended behind the other, with the heel placed firmly on the ground to target calf. Hold for 6 seconds.

Step 2: Bend back knee slightly for an Achilles stretch. Hold for 6 seconds. Shift back and forth between steps 1 and 2 three times.

FOOTWORK (HEEL RAISERS)

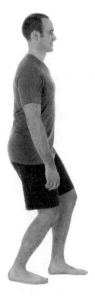

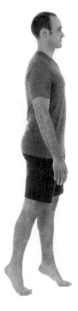

Step 1: With one foot placed slightly behind the other, bend both knees while pushing heels into the ground. Repeat 3 times.

Step 2: Contracting the ankle muscles to stop them from wobbling, raise the heels to work the feet. Completely straighten the knees. Hold this position for 6 seconds before slowly lowering heels. Return to step 1. Repeat 3 times, alternating the front leg.

LYING LEG LIFTS

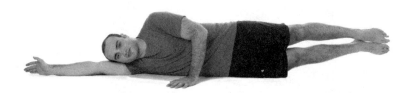

Step 1: Lying down straight, support the upper body with one arm bent and the other hand placed in front. Lie flat and raise both legs together 8 times.

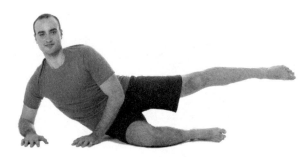

Step 2: Lift the leg with the foot pointed, focusing on continuously pulling the leg out of the hip socket and away from the body. Repeat 8 to 16 leg lifts with a pointed foot.

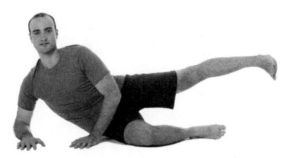

Step 3: Lift the leg with foot flexed, focusing on continuously pulling the leg out of the hip socket and away from the body. Repeat 8 to 16 leg lifts with a flexed foot.

After side leg sequence, sit up, hug your bent knees, and wiggle the hips around to release tension.

STANDING LEG LIFTS

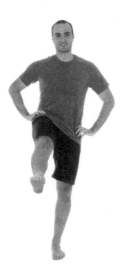

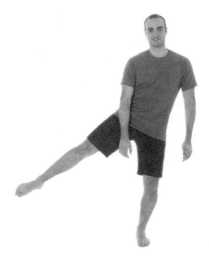

Raise and lower one leg in front of you with foot pointed, focusing on extending the leg away from you as much as possible. Keep the back straight and don't bend at the waist while lifting your leg. Do 8 to 16 leg lifts.

Raise and lower one leg to the side of your body with foot pointed, focusing on extending the leg away from you as much as possible. Rotate the knee to face the front. Do 8 to 16 side leg lifts.

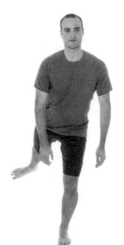

Extending your leg behind you with your bum tucked under, raise and lower the leg, focusing on pulling the leg away from the hip as much as possible. Keep the back as straight as possible and don't hunch forward. Do 8 to 16 back leg lifts.

Do 8 kicks front, side, and back, toes pointed; repeat with foot flexed; then change legs (to strengthen balance and hips). Do this for approximately 3 minutes, pulling up on the spine and keeping the back straight all the time.

PLIÉS FOR ENERGY

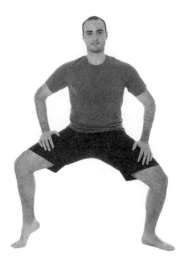

Step 1: From plié starting position, raise and lower the heel 3 times, squeezing an imaginary orange until the foot rests on the ground. These heel raisers strengthen ankles, quads, and knees.

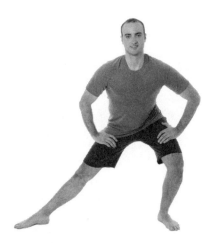

Step 2: In a plié, extend one leg until straight, keeping the other one bent and stretching the groin. Shift weight into deep side lunge.

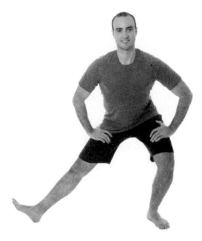

Step 3: Keep heel on the floor while flexing the ankle. Return to starting position. Repeat entire sequence 8 times, alternating sides.

CHAPTER 14

RELIEVE YOUR PAIN

Pain can come from many sources, so please check with a doctor to determine the cause of your pain. It's best to clear up any medical problems so that you can feel free to exercise as much as you want without worries. Once your doctor has ruled out anything serious, and if your pain is muscular-, joint-, or age-related, chances are the following exercises will do wonders for you.

Don't be afraid to exercise when you are in pain. The only type of pain to fear is a sharp knifelike pain, which is a warning that the body cannot tolerate what you are asking it to do, so you need to stop before you injure yourself. However, the vast majority of people in pain are afraid to move at all, assuming that it will cause them even greater pain. The irony is that movement is the best way to relieve most common pain—so move!

I am a big believer in checking with a doctor and not self-diagnosing. There are so many reasons why you are in pain.

Once a doctor gives you the all clear to exercise, the exercises I am suggesting in this chapter should help to relieve your pain. You're about to be amazed at how quickly simple exercises will relieve pain. Remember: Inactivity and a sedentary lifestyle are the number one cause of chronic pain, because they lead to muscle shrinkage and atrophy.

The human body is designed to be strong, flexible, and well balanced, and will respond rapidly to exercises. You can be in pain for years and, after just one or two workouts, start feeling relief. Pain medication is great, but it is not a cure. Medication can also exacerbate the underlying problem by masking its true severity. If the cause is

HOW TO DO PAIN RELIEF EXERCISES

This series of exercises will help relieve finger, knee, spine, hip, and calf pain. There are two stages in doing pain relief exercises:

Stage 1: Healing

Stage 1 is aimed at increasing blood flow and relieving pain immediately. In this stage, you must stay relaxed throughout the workout. Don't think of it as strengthening—think of it as healing. Keep your muscles relaxed like a rag doll! Large full-body movements done while you are relaxed help increase blood flow, which initiates healing. When muscles are contracted in strengthening mode, blood flows into them much more slowly.

Stage 2: Maintaining Relief

Stage 2 requires you to be working hard as opposed to relaxed. Only when you work hard will permanent changes happen in your muscles, allowing them to be pulled apart and strengthened simultaneously.

Stage 1 relieves you of pain; stage 2 keeps the pain from coming back. Begin stage 2 when you are no longer in pain. When you develop strength alongside flexibility, you will decompress the joints permanently, thereby stopping the squeezing from occurring. Stage 2 pulls the joints apart, giving them enough space to move easily and remain well lubricated. Stage 2 prevents the grinding of bone on bone, which is the cause of pain!

Get ready to be amazed at the pain-relieving power of your own body!

atrophy or shrinking muscles that are compressing your joints, the only way to permanently relieve that pain is to pull the joints apart (decompress them) through stretching and strengthening.

I call these *decompressing* exercises, as they release the compression caused by atrophy. These decompressing exercises apply to all joints from the vertebrae of the spine for relief of back pain to the hips, knees, feet, and fingers for relief of pain from arthritis and osteoporosis. Lengthening, strengthening, and rebalancing exercises are the secret to decompressing the joints to relieve pain. If the damage to your joints isn't so severe that joint replacements are necessary, these exercises will provide you with pain relief. Make sure you do them for 30 minutes daily (or on as regular a basis as you can manage). Every workout will take you closer to being pain-free!

WAIST ROTATIONS

Step 1: Stand with your legs apart and your arms straight above your head. Pull your arms as high as possible, until you feel your spine being stretched.

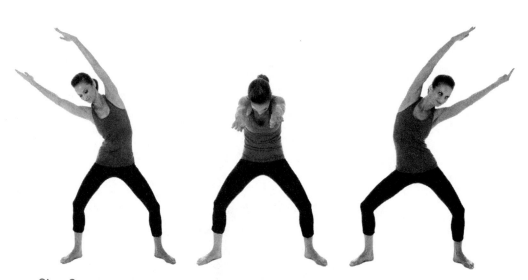

Step 2: Imagine that you are drawing a semicircle with your arms and upper body. Slowly bend sideways, still pulling your arms diagonally upward, and then continue drawing the semicircle as you move past the front and to the other side. Finish in the starting position with both arms reaching toward the ceiling. Repeat the semicircle going in the other direction. Do 4 to 6 semicircles, alternating sides.

Tip: This movement relieves back and hip pain.

ARM EXERCISES

As you do this sequence, keep the shoulders down and don't move them from steps 1 to 4.

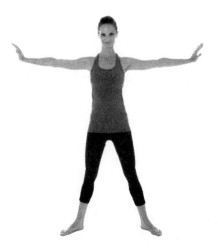

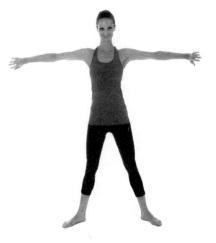

Step 1: Extend arms out toward the wall with elbows straight and hands flexed. Imagine that you are pushing a heavy weight downward as you do 8 slow pumps downward.

Step 2: Rotate arm position backward, pumping arms backward against an imaginary weight. Do 8 slow pumps backward.

Tip: These exercises help relieve pain in shoulders and fingers and are great for relieving arthritis or after a long day at the office.

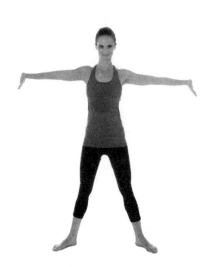

Step 3: Rotate arm position with the wrists pointing upward. Pump arms upward against an imaginary weight. Do 8 slow pumps upward.

Repeat steps 1, 2, and 3 two to four times.

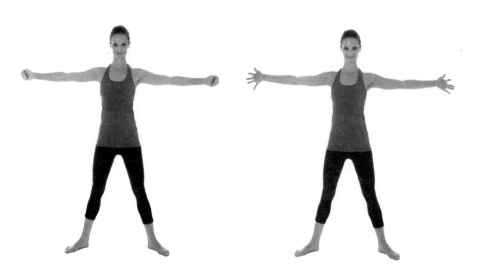

Step 4: Keep your arms extended sideways and pretend you are throwing a ball toward the front. Throw a ball at least 32 times.

CHAIR WORK FOR HIPS

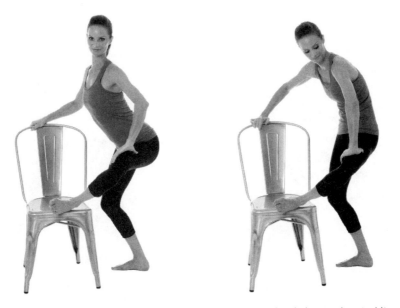

Place one foot on the seat of the chair while keeping both knees bent. Alternate between arching the back and rounding the back. This sequence of arching and tucking under is a hip and lower spine stretch that will relieve pressure and increase the mobility of your spine and improve your posture. Slowly repeat the spinal motion 3 or 4 times.

CHAIR STRETCH FOR THE PSOAS

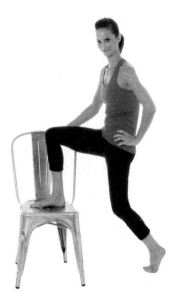

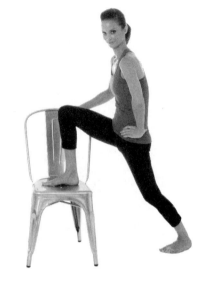

Step 1: Place the foot flat on the chair. Bend the back knee while raising the back heel and shifting the full weight of the body forward. Tuck your tailbone under until you cannot tuck under any more. Hold it there as you do step 2.

Step 2: Keeping the tailbone tucked under, slowly try to drive the standing heel into the ground. This will stretch the psoas, an important antiaging muscle. (A tight psoas is a major cause of back pain.)

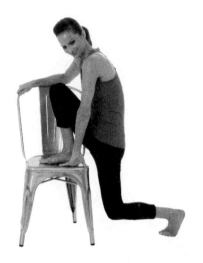

Step 3: Keeping the tailbone tucked under, carefully lower the standing leg's knee toward the floor. Keep the weight of the body on the seat of the chair. Keep moving, and the moment you go as deep as you can, immediately return to the starting position. This will stretch the quadriceps. *Never* hold these quadriceps stretches, as that would put unnecessary strain on the knee as well as overworking the quad.

Repeat steps 1, 2, and 3 three times with each leg before alternating legs.

HAMSTRING, SPINE, AND IT BAND STRETCH

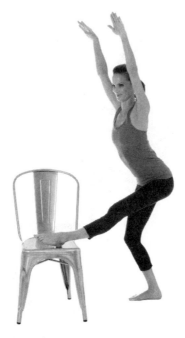

Step 1: Place the leg on the chair, trying to keep the knee straight. Bend the standing leg instead of the leg that is on the chair. Bend forward, keeping the spine straight, extending both arms over the leg, and reach one arm at a time over the leg. Keep the leg on the chair as you are reaching forward, alternating arms for 30 seconds, 5 seconds per arm.

Modification: If you cannot keep the knee straight, feel free to bend it.

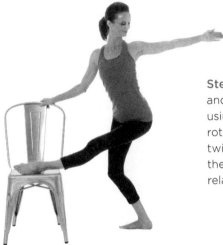

Step 2: Hold the chair with the back hand and twist the spine in opposition to the chair, using the outside arm to assist in the spine rotation. Deep-breathe in this position and twist a little farther in the exhale portion of the breath. Hold the rotation for 5 seconds, relax, and repeat 3 times.

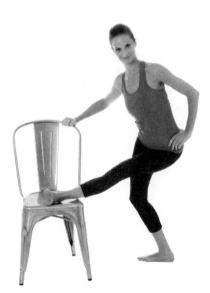

Step 3: Keeping the leg on the chair as straight as possible, drop the hip toward the chair as you flex your foot. You will feel an uncomfortable pull on the outside of your knee, which is the IT band being pulled. Move gently into and out of this stretch for about 30 seconds.

Repeat steps 1, 2, and 3 on the other leg.

LONG ADDUCTOR STRETCH

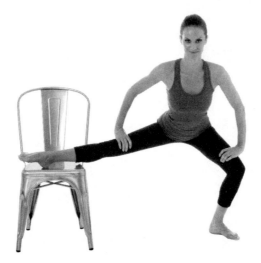

Put your leg on the chair, bend the supporting leg, and bend slightly forward. Slowly rotate the raised leg internally until you feel a stretch in your inner leg. Each person feels this stretch at a different place, so keep moving around until you feel your inner leg muscles being pulled. Once you find the stretch, move into and out of it. Do this for a maximum time of 20 seconds per leg. This exercise helps relieve hip pain.

CALF AND SOLEUS

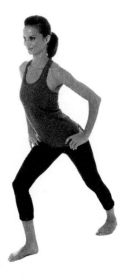 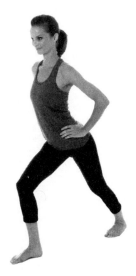

Step 1: Place one leg behind, keeping its knee straight and the heel pressing into the ground. This will stretch the long muscle of the calf. Hold this stretch for about 6 seconds, then shift into step 2.

Step 2: Bend the back knee and tuck the bum under, still keeping the heel flat on the ground. This will stretch the short muscle of the calf. Hold this stretch for about 6 seconds, and then repeat step 1. Alternate 3 times between steps 1 and 2.

PSOAS, QUADRICEPS, AND HAMSTRING STRETCH

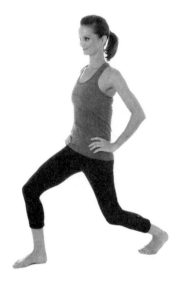

Step 1: Bend knee and lift the heel, tucking the tailbone under. This will stretch the psoas. Hold the stretch for 6 to 8 seconds, then immediately do step 2.

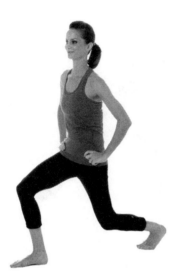

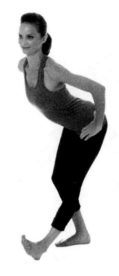

Step 2: Lower the bent knee toward the ground to stretch the quadriceps. Hold the stretch for 6 to 8 seconds. Repeat steps 1 and 2 before doing step 3.

Step 3: Extend the back leg in front, keeping the foot flexed. Bend forward, keeping your spine completely straight as you gently sway your hips side to side. This will give a full stretch to the hamstring muscle. Take 5 seconds for each hip sway and repeat 4 to 6 slow side-to-side sways.

STRETCH FOR TIGHT SHOULDERS

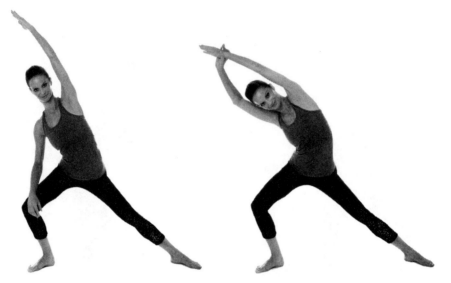

Step 1: Do a diagonal bend in a side lunge. Be sure not to raise the hip. Stretch for 6 seconds.

Step 2: Grab your wrist and pull your arm as much as possible, feeling the stretch into your ribs and down your side. Stretch for 6 seconds.

Tip: This stretch provides great upper body and shoulder pain relief.

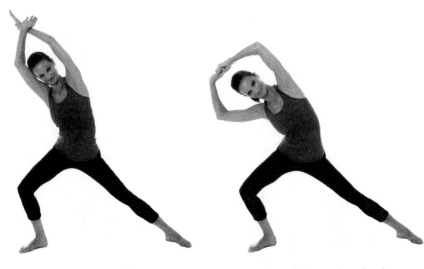

Step 3: With the lower arm, carefully press your extended arm very gently backward. This will slightly stretch the chest and shoulder muscles. Stretch for 6 seconds.

Step 4: Hold your hands above your head, making a sort of hat shape as you bend farther sideways. Stretch for 6 seconds.

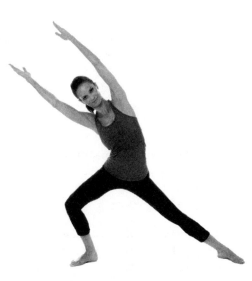

Step 5: Release the hands and straighten the arms. This will stretch spine and shoulder joints. Stretch for 6 seconds.

Repeat steps 1 to 5 on the other side, then alternate sides several times.

PLIÉS FOR KNEE PAIN RELIEF

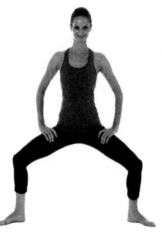 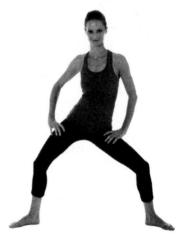

To prepare for a plié, place the legs in a wide stance with feet slightly turned out. Bend the knees into a plié, keeping them in line with the ankles. Imagine you are against a wall so that you keep your back straight.

Step 1: Shift your hips from one side to the next for a minimum of 8 times. Move slowly in order to feel the maximum stretching in your hips.

Tip: If you have tight hips, lean slightly forward to maintain balance. Many people are afraid to open their legs as Sahra is doing here. Try to get the same width as hers, as long as you have zero pain. Bend your knees until you actually sense pain, and then stop. Doing pliés this way should rapidly relieve you of chronic knee pain.

Tips: To protect the knees, keep them in line with the ankles. If you want to increase difficulty, bend into a deeper plié. Never hold a plié move even very slightly. The constant movement will increase blood flow and lubrication of the joints.

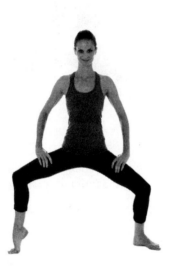

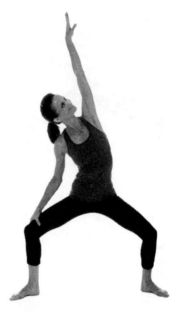

Step 2: Lift one heel off the ground to stretch the shin muscles. This will help relieve ankle, foot, and knee pain. Repeat 3 times before changing to the other foot.

Step 3: Remain in the plié and do the following arm sequence, which will work your torso in addition to your legs. Lift one arm to the ceiling, reaching up as high as possible. This will stretch your ribs and strengthen your abs while decompressing the knees.

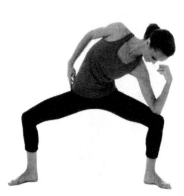

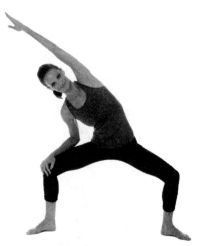

Imagine that you are pulling your arm downward, putting your elbow on your knee. This will stretch the opposite side of your body.

Finish this sequence with a deep side stretch. Repeat step 3 four times on each side before moving to step 4.

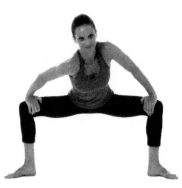

Step 4: Remain in the plié position; bend forward, keeping the spine straight; and press the knees open one at a time, to stretch the groin. Alternate knees at least 4 times.

SHOULDER BLAST SEQUENCE

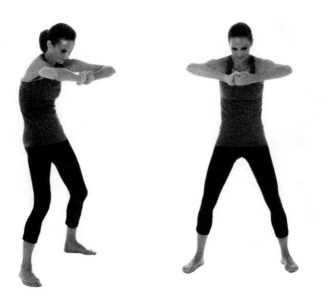

Step 1: Start with spine rounded, tail tucked under, and hands clasped in front of your body. Try to pull the hands apart, feeling a very pleasant stretching sensation in the shoulders and upper back. Technical note: Make sure you lift the shoulders during this stretch. Stretch for 6 seconds.

Tip: This is everyone's favorite feel-good exercise to relieve shoulder pain.

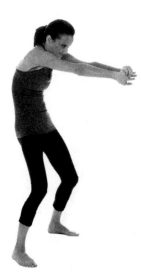

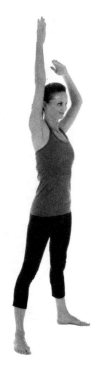

Step 2: With hands still clasped, gently press them toward the front. You should feel an additional stretch in upper back and shoulders. Stretch for 6 to 10 seconds.

Step 3: Lift one arm as high as possible toward the ceiling; this will stretch the muscles on one side of the spine. Make sure you lower the opposite shoulder in order to be able to release the muscles along the spine. Stretch for 6 seconds.

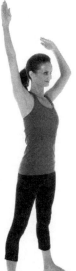

Step 4: Once you've extended your arm as high as you can, press it backward in order to stretch the pectoral muscles. This will improve your posture and relieve shoulder pain. Stretch for 3 seconds.

Repeat steps 3 and 4 with the other arm.

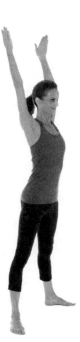

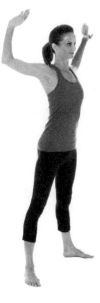

Step 5: Raise both arms above your head. Stretch for 3 seconds.

Step 6: With lots of resistance, slowly stretch the arms behind you for 6 seconds.

Repeat steps 1 to 6 at least 4 times to relieve back and shoulder pain.

CHAPTER 15

ENHANCE YOUR BALANCE

Don't forget that if we do nothing, every decade we can potentially lose between 7 and 8 percent of our cells, including nerve cells! This fact has tremendous consequences for our ability to maintain strong balance reflexes.

As we get older, it seems perfectly natural and instinctive to reach for a wall or banister, or the arm of a friend, to keep ourselves upright. Like every other aspect of aging, our loss of balance slowly creeps up on us. But like every other capability, balance is something we can maintain and improve, and we don't have to accept its loss as an inevitable part of aging.

Infants teach themselves to walk by testing the limits of their balance reflexes and pushing themselves outside their comfort zone. This forces the nerves to shoot messages into the muscles, directing them to hold the infant upright. After a few falls, the muscles get the hang of things and do hold the child upright!

To maintain our balance, we have to replicate this self-education process, forcing our nerve cells to wake up and stabilize our muscles. Nerve cells, like muscle cells, atrophy through disuse. They need to be regularly used to be maintained. We need to challenge our balance reflexes by means of an exercise that is difficult to do without losing our balance. Don't think of this as a strengthening exercise; think of it as a "deliberately falling off balance" exercise!

The exercise is aimed at stimulating your balance reflexes. It is vitally important that you do not hold on to any support while doing the movements. Like an infant, you have to make your balance reflexes shoot the message to wake up into your muscles. If you are nervous about falling over, stand near a wall so that at any time you will be able to immediately reach for it. (But try to reach for the wall as seldom as possible.) Though at first you may find the exercise difficult and taxing, your balance should improve quickly. It definitely won't get worse!

DRAWING THE ALPHABET

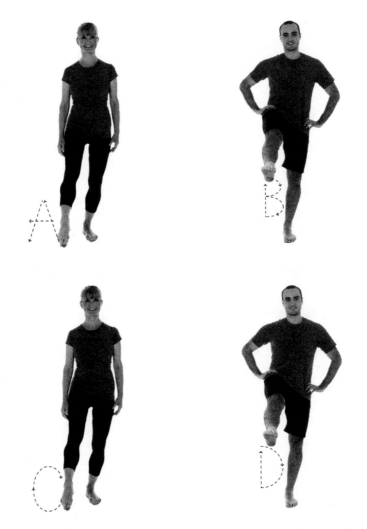

The best balance exercise I know is to stand on one leg while drawing the alphabet with the other one. Start slowly and go as far up the alphabet as you can before changing legs.

The objective is to eventually be able to stand on one leg and write the whole alphabet from A to Z before changing legs. Then do it again so that you draw the alphabet twice with both legs. It might take a few weeks before you are able to draw it twice through at one session. It's fun!

Tip: This exercise stimulates your balance reflexes.

CHAPTER 16

IMPROVE YOUR MOBILITY

Sometimes, after a particularly long movie-watching binge, even young adults can feel stiff when they stand up from the sofa. Or athletes who've overtrained cannot comfortably bend down to sit on the floor—let alone get up again. And it's very common for people who lead a sedentary life to have trouble getting into and out of a car. To make matters worse, the degree of difficulty getting into and out of a car tends to increase with every additional pound of body weight. The reason it is difficult getting into and out of a car, or sitting on and standing up from a sofa, or getting onto or off the floor is that the muscles have become weak from lack of use and are already in various stages of atrophy.

An adult body is heavy. Try lifting a full-grown adult or even a child and you will find that it is a heavy load. You need strength to lift the weight of your body and if your muscles are weak, it is exhausting and very difficult to get out of or into a car.

Muscles are designed to atrophy when you don't use them and when you are sedentary—your muscles literally shrink. But don't panic! You can do a lot to change that, as long as you are prepared to do 30 minutes of exercise every day. The best way to get into the habit is to do your exercises when you wake up, before eating or washing. They'll be done before you know it!

If you've never made exercise a priority, there comes a time when your personal quality of life and the effect your health issues have on the people closest to you begin to dictate every other decision you make. Having weak muscles is bad for your health and a huge stress on the people around you. If you have trouble getting into and out of a car, eventually you will require assistance; and heave-hoing a heavy person often injures the person who is assisting. I have seen an astonishing number of unnecessary injuries suffered by family members, nurses, and other caregivers in helping weak patients to turn over in bed or get off a chair.

Gaining strength by exercising on a regular basis is an act of love toward those people who care about you. Maybe you're not there yet; maybe you're a young mom who has all she can do just chasing her kids around and you don't exercise for yourself. Maybe you get worn out when you take your kids to the roller rink. Take a good look at the older woman struggling to get out of her car—she is you in 20 (or 10!) years, unless you act now!

We all need full-body strength and flexibility, particularly in the legs, hips, and lower back, to be able to be independent and move around easily.

So let's start solving the problem with a few exercises. The best way to begin strengthening all the muscles involved in getting into and out of a car or standing up on roller skates is to stand up and sit down as rapidly as possible. Repeat that 10 times in a row and then do it again a few hours later. Do this sitting-standing sequence several times a day; it is an easy way to quickly strengthen the muscles and joints in your hips, back, and knees. If you are sedentary, it will most likely be totally exhausting to do for the first day or so—and you might be able to do only two or three repetitions of getting up and down in a row. But trust me—your body is craving strengthening movements and will respond really rapidly. Before a week is over you will be moving much faster, much more easily, and with much less effort.

Once you have made some progress, add some of the exercises listed here. The pliés will strengthen your quad and hip muscles, and the seated groin stretch will add flexibility to your hips. When exiting a car or pulling ourselves up from the floor on roller skates, we need to rotate the spine; the windmill stretch will increase both flexibility and strength along the spine, making the turning movement easier and more efficient. The side-to-side lunges will strengthen the legs and hips, and feet, as well as the spine.

They will also add flexibility to the inner leg and the groin—which will really help your skating as well as help you as you step out of the car. And the arm figure 8 exercises will add flexibility to the upper body, so that the twisting movement the body automatically makes will be more fluid when we are entering and exiting a car.

Do these exercises at least once a day; I suggest you do them every morning and several times a day. If you feel a little nauseated the first few times you do these exercises, or even a little dizzy, don't worry. This dizziness is often caused by the toxins being flushed out, as your blood circulates more efficiently and oxygen is delivered to your cells. Be as lazy as you want at first, as long as you move a bit to stimulate blood flow. Every time you do the exercises you can work a little bit harder. The best way to build up your muscles and strength is slowly and progressively. Pretty soon you will feel like a new person!

CLOCK

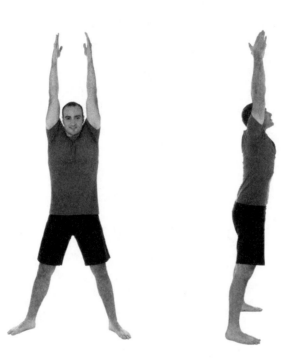

Step 1: Stand upright with arms extended straight above head, reaching up as high as possible. Notice in the side view how straight the spine is.

Tip: This exercise helps develop spine and core strength and mobility.

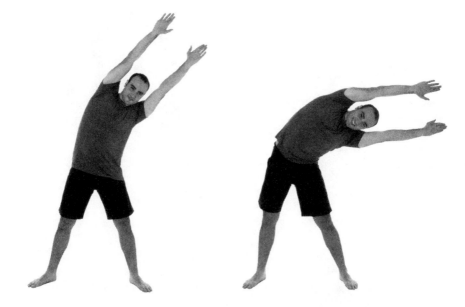

Step 2: Bend sideways, pulling up and away from the body with as much strength as possible, keeping the arms close together.

Step 3: Slowly bend deeper. Take 6 seconds to bend sideways and 6 seconds to straighten to starting position. This exercise will strengthen the spine and increase mobility of the torso. Repeat steps 2 and 3 four times, alternating sides each time.

PLIÉS FOR HIP, KNEE, AND TORSO MOBILITY

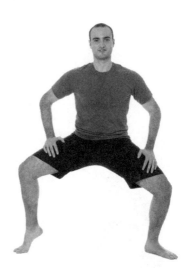

Step 1: Raise and lower the heel 3 times, squeezing an imaginary orange until the foot is flat on the ground. These heel raisers strengthen ankles, quads, and knees.

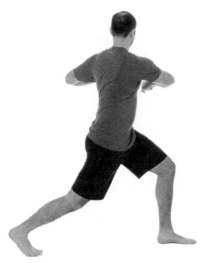

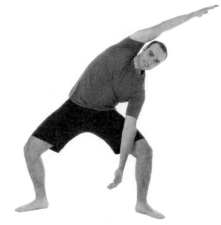

Step 2: From a basic plié position, twist on the spine, rotating toward the back of the room. This will strengthen and stretch the back and hip muscles. Remain in the plié position as you alternate sides 8 times.

Step 3: Remaining in the basic plié position, bend side to side. This will strengthen the core muscles.

SEATED GROIN STRETCH

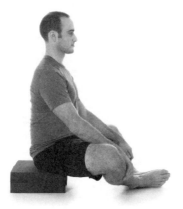

Sit with legs bent and feet touching, keeping the back straight. Notice that James is sitting on two raisers. Many people need to sit on a raiser when doing groin stretches; it helps to straighten the spine and target the correct groin muscles.

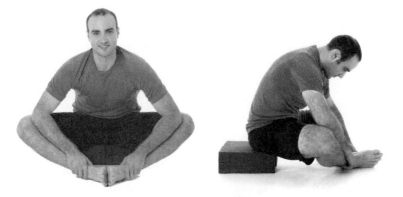

Step 1: Bending forward, gently push the knees downward, using the elbows to press down on the knees. Press downward for roughly 6 seconds.

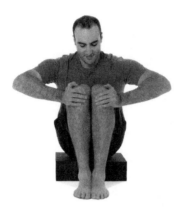 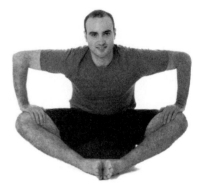

Step 2: Squeeze the legs together with the hands while trying to open the legs with leg muscles. Do this for 6 seconds. Quickly release the tension and go into step 3.

Step 3: Press knees downward to stretch groin. This move will assist the groin to be able to go into a much deeper groin stretch when you release the knees. Do this for 6 seconds

Repeat steps 1, 2, and 3 four times.

DEEP SIDE-TO-SIDE BENDS

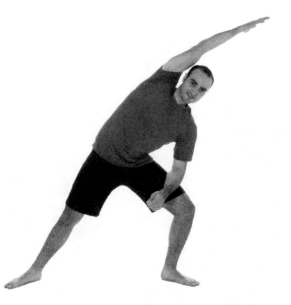

Alternate 16 slow consecutive side lunges. This exercise will help you to move more easily, whether you are playing tennis or getting into and out of a car, a bathtub, or bed.

SINGLE-ARM FIGURE 8

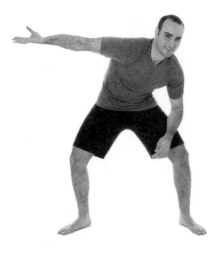

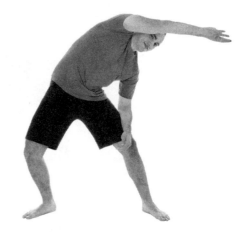

Step 1: Bend slightly forward while rounding the back. Twist an extended arm internally and begin to sweep it across the front of the body. This will stretch and increase the mobility of the upper back. Take 6 seconds to finish the slow movement, going from step 1 to step 2.

Step 2: Finish sweeping across the body in an extended diagonal reach.

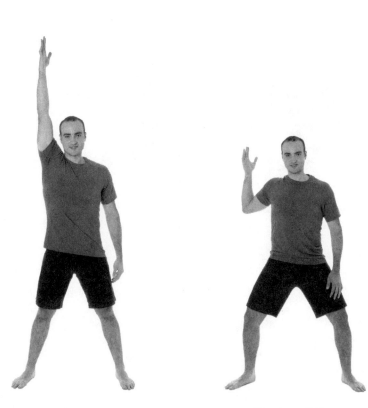

Step 3: Slowly raise the arm straight above the head while straightening the full spine and torso, taking 6 seconds to straighten up.

Step 4: Slowly pull the arms downward and prepare to begin the full rotation of the arm again.

Repeat steps 1 to 4 four times before changing sides.

SPINAL ROLLS

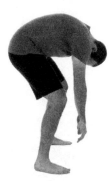

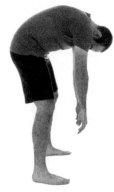

Step 1: Start by bending forward in a relaxed position with head and arms hanging down. This exercise increases the mobility of the spine.

Step 2: Roll one spinal vertebra at a time, reaching from the floor to ceiling, remaining relaxed throughout the movement.

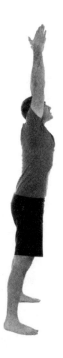

Step 3: Finish standing up tall. Note: Do not drop your weight backward as you pull the arms upward.

Repeat steps 1 to 3 four times slowly, taking 6 to 10 seconds to complete the full spinal roll.

DIAGONAL WINDMILLS

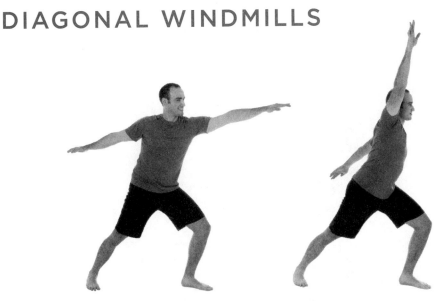

Step 1: Windmill sequences are accomplished by continuously rotating the arms from back to front, to resemble the motion of a windmill. Start in a front lunge, doing a diagonal reach toward the corner with one arm forward and the other arm behind.

Step 2: Start the windmill movement of the arms. Take 8 to 10 seconds to finish one complete windmill.

Tip: This exercise increases the range of motion of the spine.

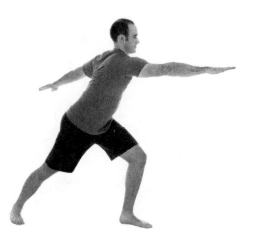

Step 3: Continue on, never stopping the rotational movement of the arms.

Do 8 slow windmills per side before changing to the other leg and other side.

HIP CLEANERS

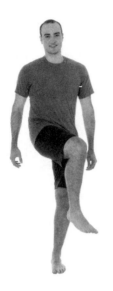

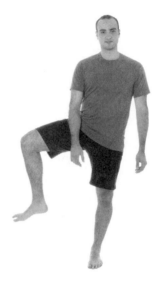

Step 1: Holding a chair or freestanding, pull the bent leg across the body to stretch the outer hip muscles.

Step 2: Open the bent leg sideways, keeping it as high as possible without lifting your hip.

Step 3: Pull the bent leg behind the body, keeping it bent and raised as high as possible.

Repeat steps 1 to 3 four or five times per leg. The aim of the hip cleaners is to clean away scar tissue in the hips and to relax the hip muscles. This will make for much easier hip movement and greater hip mobility.

Tip: This exercise increases hip mobility.

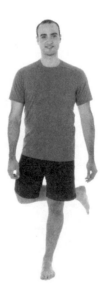

HIP STRETCH WITH KNEE BENT

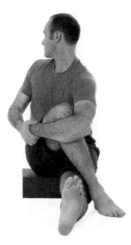

From a sitting position, embrace knee and place the foot as close to the hip as possible, making sure the foot is flat on the ground. Pull the knee into the chest. Rotate on the spine to face the back of the room. You should feel a deep hip stretch. Stretch each leg for 30 seconds.

SEATED SPINE STRETCH

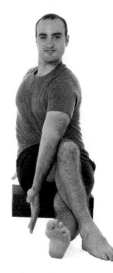

Place the foot near the calf. Keep the spine straight and cross the opposite arm over the knee. Twist the spine, using the arm as a lever. Deeply inhale, and on the exhale, try to twist the spine farther. Inhale for 5 seconds and exhale for 5 seconds. Repeat 3 times, then change sides.

Tip: This exercise increases spinal mobility.

IT BAND STRETCH
WHILE HOLDING FOOT

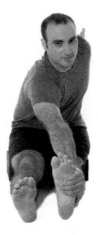

Do this IT band or knee stretch by taking the flexed foot in the opposite hand and gently pull the torso closer to the foot. If you cannot reach your foot, hold any part of your leg that you can easily reach and, as you twist your spine, pull the body forward, keeping the foot flexed. Do 15 seconds on each leg.

CHAPTER 17

PROTECT YOUR BONES

Osteoporosis is a condition in which the bones become thin and brittle, losing their density and their resiliency, and greatly increasing their risk of fracture. The severity of osteoporosis can range from mild to extreme, beginning very slowly with the pre-osteoporosis condition called osteopenia.

In its earliest stages, osteopenia is imperceptible and has no effect on our daily lives. But when osteopenia progresses to osteoporosis, the pain becomes constant and the shape of the body changes. Anyone suffering from osteoporosis, particularly anyone in its advanced stages, must be careful not to fracture a bone when exercising. Consult a doctor for permission before doing the following exercises. These exercises should help to combat osteoporosis and retard its progression at any stage.

The best course of action is preventive. Weight-bearing exercises are necessary to prevent or reverse osteoporosis by increasing bone density. You don't need to run to a gym or to a store to purchase weights—the human body itself is sufficiently heavy to safely stress our bones. The average woman in the United States weighs 165 pounds and the average man weighs 195 pounds. The average arm weighs about the same as a medium-size watermelon. That's a lot of weight to lift! Unless you particularly love lifting weights, you will never need to lift more weight than your own body.

Traditional weight training often focuses on the obvious large bones in the body while ignoring all the rest. Osteoporosis attacks all our bones, not just the biggest ones! So you have to strengthen them all, right?

The 200 bones in our body are the structure around which we are shaped. When the bones soften, the structure collapses, and we look deformed and shrunken. The point at which the spine collapses from osteoporosis is the most visible sign of the condition. In order to straighten the spine, we need to strengthen the vertebrae, the bones of the spine, by moving them in all directions—bending forward, backward, sideways, and rotationally.

Our muscles enable any movement as they lift and lower our bones. Each time we move, the bones are stressed or de-stressed. That stress stimulates and reawakens the cells, in effect strengthening them. That is what makes osteoporosis reverse.

To understand the relationship between the bones and muscles, I imagine a marionette, complete with strings. This image aptly conveys how our bones and muscles work together. Every move we make, no matter how small, requires a symphony of muscles and bones working together in harmony. As our muscles lift and lower our bodies through large and small movements, stresses are continually being put on and taken off our bones. These movements cause blood to be pumped into and out of the bones, flushing out the wasteful by-products of cell maintenance and bringing in calcium and other bone-strengthening minerals and nutrients.

Every movement, every gesture, every exercise helps to stress the bones, which in turn fight back by building stronger "walls." Our bodies have a honeycomb-like matrix that acts as a receptor to the minerals and crystals inside the walls of the bones. With osteoporosis this matrix crumbles, so there is nowhere for the minerals and crystals to be deposited. They are flushed out of the bone and the bone becomes porous and soft.

Exercise stresses the bones, helping to rebuild the crumbling matrix that is characteristic of osteoporosis. Large rotational movement pumps blood into the bones, delivering minerals and crystals with it. Once the honeycomb-like matrix is rebuilt the crystals can be deposited into the receptors on the matrix. This is how to reverse or prevent osteoporosis.

After working closely with many doctors for over 15 years, receiving many medical reports from students attesting to their personal reversal of osteoporosis, and seeing clients in my own centers reversing their osteoporosis without using weights, I now firmly believe that we do not need to use weights to reverse or prevent osteoporosis. Our own bodies provide sufficient weight to tax our muscles and bone structure. What we do need is bone-stressing exercises, whatever they are, and we need to do them on a regular basis.

I have put together a series of exercises to help prevent and reverse osteoporosis. None of the ESSENTRICS exercises should be done with external weights—any external weight could actually cause joint damage. These or similar full-body exercises should be done every day for about half an hour for the rest of your life.

ARM EXERCISES

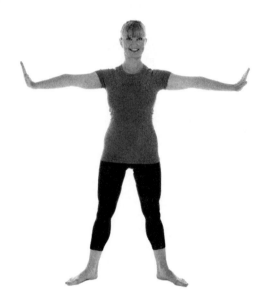

Extend arms out toward the wall with the elbows straight and hands flexed. Do 32 pumps downward against imaginary resistance to strengthen the bones of the spine and shoulders.

THROW A BALL

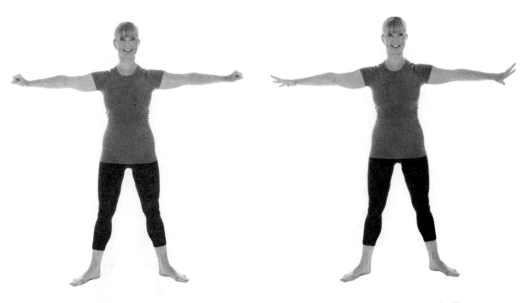

Step 1: Hold the ball!   **Step 2:** Throw the ball!

Repeat steps 1 and 2 thirty-two times to strengthen the bones of the arms and fingers.

DIAGONAL STRETCHES

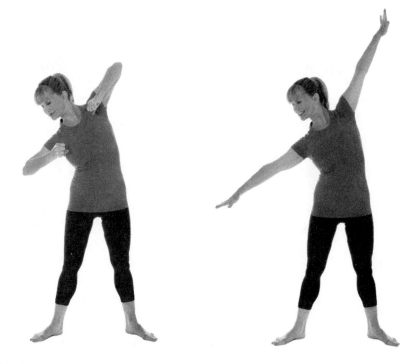

Step 1: Bend sideways as you also bend your elbows while making a tight fist. This increases blood flow when you open the fists.

Step 2: Open arms into a diagonal stretch, opening the fist at the same time. This will strengthen the bones of the spine.

MAKE A STAR

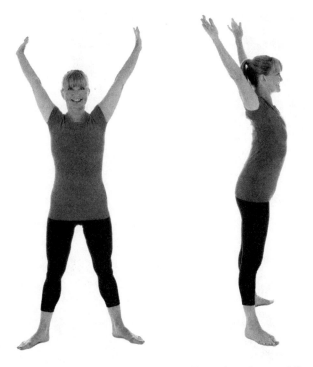

Step 1: Open both arms above the head, pulling them toward the upper back corners of the room.

Tip: This exercise strengthens the bones of the spine and shoulders.

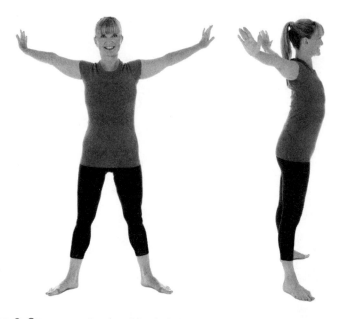

Step 2: Open arms to shoulder height, pulling arms backward.

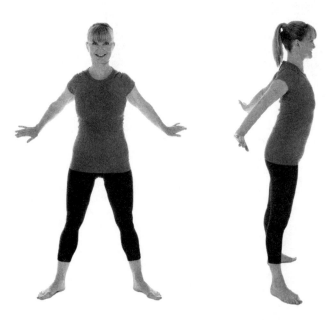

Step 3: Open arms to 45 degrees below shoulders, also pulling arms backward. Repeat steps 1 to 3 a minimum of 8 to 10 times.

Tip: Never bend backward. Keep your spine always leaning slightly forward.

FOOTWORK WITH CHAIR

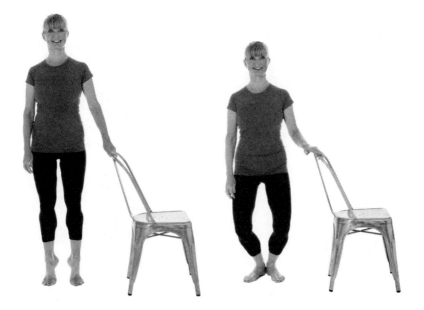

Holding on to a chair, lower and raise heels while bending and straightening the knees.

This exercise will build strong leg and foot bones. Do 32 lowerings and raisings of the heels.

FOOTWORK FOR SHINS, FEET, AND LEGS

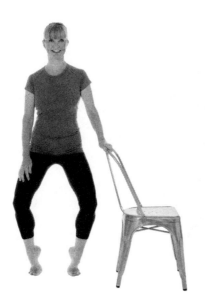

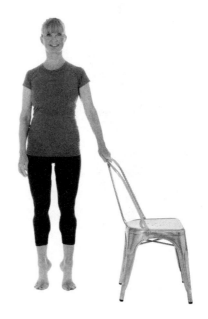

Step 1: Do a plié, lifting heels while holding a chair for balance.

Step 2: Straighten the legs.

Repeat steps 1 and 2 eight times slowly. This series will strengthen the shins, feet, and leg bones.

FOOTWORK FOR HIP AND ANKLE BONES

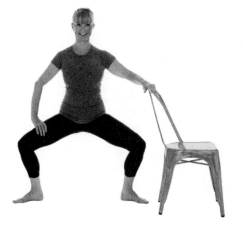 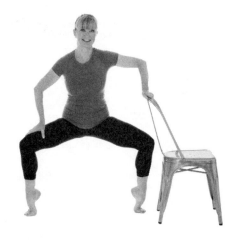

Step 1: Start with heel flat on the ground in a wide-stance plié.

Step 2: Raise heels as high as possible to deeply stretch the shins and increase the ankles' mobility.

Repeat steps 1 and 2 eight times.

HIP STRENGTHENERS

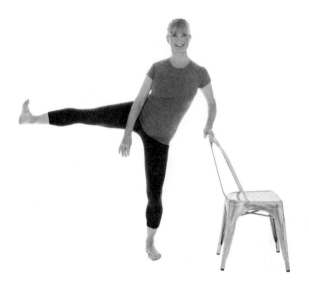

Holding a chair, flex the foot while doing 16 side kicks. This will strengthen the standing leg and hip bones.

HIP AND LEG STRENGTHENERS

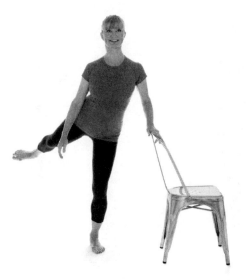

Holding a chair, flex the foot while doing 16 back kicks. This will strengthen the hip bones.

SPINE AND LEG STRENGTHENERS

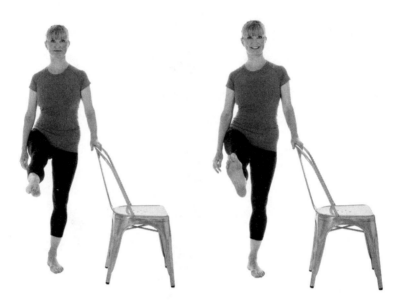

Holding a chair, do 16 front kicks with the toes pointed and repeat with the foot flexed.

Tip: Try not to move the spine. When lifting the leg, lift only with leg muscles, *not* back muscles. (Height is not important.)

CHAIR TRICEPS

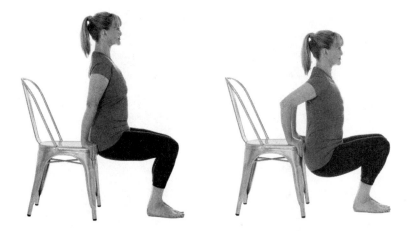

Start in a 90-degree position to the ground with hands on chair.

Slowly lower the body, staying as close to the chair as possible. Do 8 chair triceps strengtheners, rest for a few seconds, then repeat the full exercise 4 times.

Tip: This exercise uses the full weight of your body to stress the arm and shoulder bones.

STANDING LEG KICKS

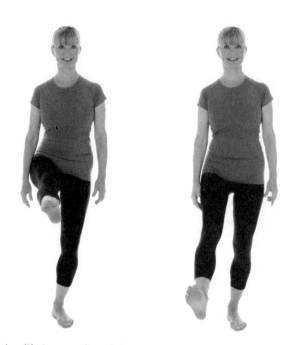

Kick leg in front with toes pointed, keeping back completely straight. Contract your abdominals throughout the entire exercise. Don't forget to breathe even though you're holding your stomach tight! Repeat 32 times per side, then repeat with foot flexed.

STANDING HIP STRENGTHENERS

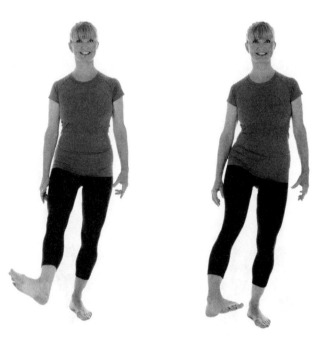

Rotate the leg internally and externally 8 times for each leg to increase blood flow into the hips.

SIDE AND CEILING REACHES FOR STRENGTHENING THE SPINE

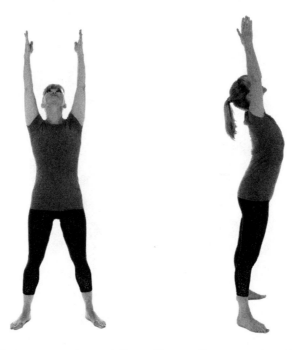

Step 1: Reach your arms toward the ceiling, pulling up as much as possible to strengthen the large and small muscles of the spine. *Do not bend backward.*

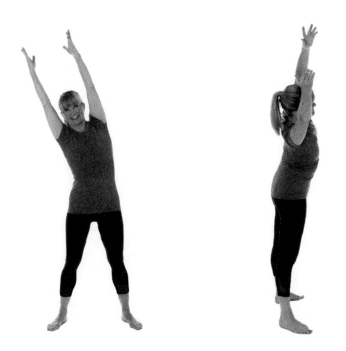

Step 2: Bend torso sideways, keeping abs tight and pulling up as much as possible. Take 6 seconds to bend sideways and 6 seconds to return to starting position. Repeat 4 to 6 times, alternating sides each time.

THE POWER OF LIFE

Life is a powerful force that does not surrender quietly. Life fights for every second of survival. Yet time moves steadily and slowly forward. We have to keep vigilant and not let ourselves age prematurely, despite the movement of time. I've shown you that you do have a choice, provided you commit yourself to daily exercise. Time never stops, so neither can we.

To remain feeling youthful, we must choose to prevent cell death.

To remain feeling youthful, we must choose to prevent atrophy.

To remain feeling youthful, we must choose to prevent poor posture.

Doing nothing is a sin of omission rather than commission. Doing nothing is a choice to let your body decay before its time. Doing something is the choice to stay vital, healthy, and youthful.

We are born with DNA that gives us a vague expiration date. But what we are *not* born with is the quality of that life we will have between birth and death. The quality of our lives is where free will and the element of choice come in.

I have shown you that we have control over how rapid the process leading toward death will be. I have shown you that through regular exercise you can maintain good posture, high energy, strength, and mobility. You have control over how much you will suffer from fatigue and chronic pain or how wonderful you will feel. The control rests in your choice to be sedentary or active.

I have shown you that without regular exercise, you are almost guaranteed to age rapidly and painfully. Atrophy is painful; arthritis is painful; weakness is exhausting. We have two clear choices, action and inaction—there is no third choice. There is no putting off the choice till you feel like making it. All you are "putting off" is your chance of having a vital, exciting, energized time well into your twilight years.

The pace of time is calm and steady; it is not desperate or frantic. We don't need to exercise frantically to keep up with the pace of time: 30 minutes of gentle exercise each day will keep time at bay. Half an hour every day is all you need to do if you want to be able to dress and undress yourself without assistance, enjoy an active relationship with friends and family, and not tire easily during the day. Half an hour a day is all you need to keep your muscles strong and pain-free. Most of us are not asking a great deal; what we are asking is to feel young rather than old, healthy rather than unhealthy.

To slow down and reverse the signs of aging requires us to show a minimal amount of discipline by participating in half an hour of daily exercise. That's it!

If we want good posture, we have to maintain strong flexible back muscles. Without regular exercise our muscles are programmed to atrophy and become tight. If that happens, we won't have the strength to maintain good posture.

If we want to have energy, we have to stoke the fires of the mitochondria to give us energy; if we don't exercise, calories aren't burned to give us energy and we will feel tired all the time.

After reading this book you know what's happening inside your body to make you age. You also know what you can do to prevent your body from aging. You now have a choice.

I am here not only to educate you about the choice but also to encourage you to choose the path of greater health. I've chosen to be active and I am thrilled with the way my life is turning out. I'm not naive; I know that staying active doesn't mean I will never get sick. I've had my share of major illnesses and broken bones, so I know what they are about. Because of that experience, I know I can live through them and come out even stronger. Being active means that I have a good chance of fast recovery; probability is on my side. It also means that I will feel healthy and vital well into my senior years. Being active means that I can enjoy my life. I can enjoy my daughter and my friends. I can look forward to traveling. I can look forward to every year with the expectation of a new adventure. I am no longer waiting for "old age" to happen to me. I know now how I can have a fun life until I die. And that is what I am doing.

What more could anyone ask for?

As I watched my father struggle to stay alive in his final months, I was struck with the knowledge that all of us have the same powerful force of life coursing through our veins.

All we have to do is activate that force of life within us, and that force will respond a thousandfold.

The smallest movements will turn on the mitochondria and start the fires of life!

The smallest movements will start the fountain of youth flowing throughout our veins!

Life is programmed to live.
Life is created to live.
Life does not surrender easily.
We can be strong
If we choose to be strong.
We can be energetic
If we choose to be energetic.
We can be pain-free
If we choose to be pain-free.
We can be independent
If we choose to be independent.
But if we choose all that, we must choose to move.
We must choose to exercise!

ACKNOWLEDGMENTS

Although the actual writing of a book is very solitary, the truth is that it impossible to write a book of this nature without a great deal of assistance. Some authors do all the work and rightfully should receive all the credit. However, in the case of *Aging Backwards*, there are many people who deserve acknowledgment and thanks for their valuable contributions.

There have been many editors for this manuscript but the first brave soul to clean up the book was Philip Clark, who gets special credit for taking a sharp scalpel to my rambling text and turning it into beautiful prose.

A book of this nature requires hours of research and acquisition of legal rights for the different scientific studies and charts that we have quoted and used throughout the book. Lynda Whyte, Melissa Tran, and Annabel Tory, all very talented and remarkable women, have worked side by side over many months to acquire the needed material.

I'd also like to mention that Annabel's impressive organizational skills made a very complex photo shoot seem simple and easy. I would be remiss not to thank Annabel for taking over the official editing scalpel for cutting more repeated thoughts and overlong sentences. And I also want to thank Sydney Pierce at HarperWave for her hard work making sure every photo and everything else was sewn up tight and ready for publication.

Finding models for photography can be easy—but finding the *right* model is not so easy. We were very lucky that James Gadon agreed to model for the photos in the book. James is a former hockey player and recent Classical Stretch/ESSENTRICS instructor. I think he did an outstanding job in clearly demonstrating the exercises in this book.

Writing a book, even a very good book, is one thing, but actually being able to introduce it to major publishers is a whole other obstacle. I have noticed that authors tend to gush about their agents and now I know why. A good agent is indeed worth gushing about, and Ryan Fisher is tops in his field. I would like to thank my lucky stars that I met Ryan, who had faith in *Aging Backwards* and the ability to introduce it to the correct people. I am very grateful for his patience and encouragement and mostly for his hard work and intelligence in guiding *Aging Backwards* into the hands of HarperWave, the American and worldwide publisher, and Random House, its Canadian publisher.

Now I am tempted to start an embarrassing amount of thanks and gushing. What would a book do without publishers who understand the needs and tastes of their readers? I am so grateful to both my publishers: Julie Will, executive editor at HarperWave, the worldwide publisher of *Aging Backwards*; and Anne Collins at Random House, the Canadian publisher. Julie believed in the book so strongly that she recruited the ghost-writing talents of Mariska van Aalst. Between the two of them, they took on the role of book doctor and rewrote the book so that you, the reader, could easily enjoy and access the knowledge on its pages. Thanks to Mariska and Julie, it is a pleasure to read. Again, I must gush, thanking Anne Collins, vice president of Random House Canada, not only for publishing *Aging Backwards* in Canada but for also actually doing the workouts on a daily basis and seeing firsthand how these exercises have helped her age backwards. There is no greater honor for me than to have these three amazing women in my corner.

Finally, I'd like to thank my daughter, Sahra, and my mother for their love, encouragement, and support throughout the long years of developing ESSENTRICS. Being able to share its success with them has made the experience so much more enjoyable. ESSENTRICS really is the child of three generations of Esmonde-White women. I am so grateful that Sahra finally persuaded me to write this book. Over these years, she has witnessed how inspired both friends and strangers were after hearing me lecture on *Aging Backwards*. It took her a long time to convince me, but now I am extremely grateful that she never stopped pushing. Sahra has always been my greatest cheerleader, believing that this was a story that would help and inspire many people to live healthier and happier lives.

NOTES

1. E. T. Poehlman, C. L. Melby, and S. F. Badylak. "Relation of age and physical exercise status on metabolic rate in younger and older healthy men," *J Gerontol*, March 1991: 46(2):B54–58. PubMed PMID: 1997564.

2. R. E. Van Pelt, P. P. Jones, K. P. Davy, C. A. Desouza, H. Tanaka, B. M. Davy, and D. R. Seals. "Regular exercise and the age-related decline in resting metabolic rate in women," *J Clin Endocrinol Metab*, October 1997: 82(10):3208–12. PubMed PMID: 9329340.

3. R. E. Van Pelt, F. A. Dinneno, D. R. Seals, and P. P. Jones. "Age-related decline in RMR in physically active men: relation to exercise volume and energy intake," *Am J Physiol Endocrinol Metab*, September 2001: 281(3):E633–39. PubMed PMID: 11500320.

4. M. A. Tarnopolsky. "ACSM Exchange Lecture: Exercise as a countermeasure for aging—from mice to humans," American Medical Society for Sports Medicine 23rd annual meeting, April 6, 2014, New Orleans, http://www.amssm.org/Content/pdf%20files/2014_AM-Brochure .pdf; http://well.blogs.nytimes.com/2014/04/16/younger-skin-through-exercise/.

5. A. P. Wroblewski, F. Amati, M. A. Smiley, B. Goodpaster, and V. Wright, "Chronic exercise preserves lean muscle mass in masters athletes," Department of Orthopaedic Surgery, University of Pittsburgh, Pittsburgh, PA, *The Physician and Sportsmedicine*, April 25, 2011: 171(8), web.

6. E. Weiderpass. "Lifestyle and cancer risk," *J Prev Med Public Health*, November 2010: 43(6):459–71. doi: 10.3961/jpmph.2010.43.6.459. PubMed PMID: 21139406.

7. R. F. Hamman, R. R. Wing, S. L. Edelstein, J. M. Lachin, G. A. Bray, L. Delahanty, M. Hoskin, A. M. Kriska, E. J. Mayer-Davis, X. Pi-Sunyer, J. Regensteiner, B. Venditti, and J. Wylie-Rosett. "Effect of weight loss with lifestyle intervention on risk of diabetes," *Diabetes Care*, September 2006: 29(9):2102–7. PubMed PMID: 16936160; PubMed Central PMCID: PMC1762038.

8. M. J. Stampfer, F. B. Hu, J. E. Manson, E. B. Rimm, and W. C. Willett. "Primary prevention of coronary heart disease in women through diet and lifestyle," *N Engl J Med*, July 6, 2000: 343(1):16–22. PubMed PMID: 10882764.

9. A. Wroblewski, F. Amati, M. Smiley, B. Goodpaster, and V. Wright. "Chronic exercise preserves lean muscle mass in masters athletes," *The Physician and Sports Medicine*, 2011: 39(3), 172–78.

10. See http://www.ncbi.nlm.nih.gov/pubmed/16677099.

11. See http://commonhealth.wbur.org/2013/03/minutes-exercise-longer-life; S. C. Moore, A. V. Patel, C. E. Matthews, A. Berrington de Gonzalez, Y. Park, H. A. Katki, M. S. Linet, E. Weiderpass, K. Visvanathan, K. J. Helzlsouer, M. Thun, S. M. Gapstur, P. Hartge, and I. M. Lee. "Leisure time physical activity of moderate to vigorous intensity and mortality: a large pooled cohort analysis," *PLoS Med*, 2012: 9(11):e1001335. doi: 10.1371/journal.pmed.1001335. Epub November 6, 2012. PubMed PMID: 23139642; PubMed Central PMCID: PMC3491006.

12. A. R. Brooks-Wilson. "Genetics of healthy aging and longevity," *Human Genetics*, December 2013: 132, Issue 12, pp. 1323-38.

13. NIH. "Mitochondria: cellular power plants. Chapter 1: An owner's guide to the cell: inside the cell," http://publications.nigms.nih.gov/insidethecell/chapter1.html#6.

14. "Tocris bioscience." *Apoptosis.* http://www.tocris.com/pharmacologicalBrowser.php?ItemId=187886#.U2eGRyhr204

15. A. G. Renehan, C. Booth, and C. S. Potten. "What is apoptosis, and why is it important?" *BMJ*, June 23, 2001: 322(7301):1536-38. Review. PubMed PMID: 11420279; PubMed Central PMCID: PMC1120576.

16. T. Finkel. "Telomeres and mitochondrial function." *Circ Res*, April 15, 2011: 108(8):903–4. doi: 10.1161/RES.0b013e31821bc2d8. PubMed PMID: 21493920; PubMed Central PMCID: PMC3747515.

17. J. C. Kovacic, P. Moreno, V. Hachinski, E. G. Nabel, and V. Fuster. "Cellular senescence, vascular disease, and aging: part 1 of a 2-part review," *Circulation*, April 19, 2011: 123(15):1650–60. doi: 10.1161/CIRCULATIONAHA.110.007021. Review. PubMed PMID: 21502583.

18. Renehan et al. "What is apoptosis, and why is it important?"

19. NIH, "The last chapter: cell aging and death. Chapter 5: Inside the cell." http://publications.nigms.nih.gov/insidethecell/chapter5.html

20. D. F. Dai, P. S. Rabinovitch, and Z. Ungvari. "Mitochondria and cardiovascular aging," *Circ Res*, April 13, 2012: 110(8):1109-24. doi: 10.1161/CIRCRESAHA.111.246140. Review. PubMed PMID: 22499901; PubMed Central PMCID: PMC3867977.

21. T. Finkel. "Telomeres and mitochondrial function," *Circ Res*, April 15, 2011: 108(8): 903–4. doi: 10.1161/RES.0b013e31821bc2d8. PubMed PMID: 21493920; PubMed Central PMCID: PMC3747515.

22. NIH, "The last chapter: cell aging and death."

23. A. M. Molnar, S. Servais, M. Guichardant, M. Lagarde, D. Macedo, L. Pereira-Da-Silva, B. Sibille, and R. Favier. "Mitochondrial H2O2 production is reduced with acute and chronic eccentric exercise in rat skeletal muscle," *Antioxid Redox Signal*, March–April 2006: 8(3–4):548-58. PubMed PMID: 16677099.

24. R. David. "Ageing: mitochondria and telomeres come together," *Nat Rev Mol Cell Biol*, April 2011: 12(4):204. doi: 10.1038/nrm3082. Epub March 16, 2011. PubMed PMID: 21407239.

25. I. R. Lanza and K. S. Nair. "Mitochondrial function as a determinant of life span," *Pflugers Arch*, January 2010: 459(2):277-89. doi: 10.1007/s00424-009-0724-5. Epub September 11, 2009. Review. PubMed PMID: 19756719; PubMed Central PMCID: PMC2801852.

26. A. T. Ludlow, J. B. Zimmerman, S. Witkowski, J. W. Hearn, B. D. Hatfield, and S. M. Roth. "Relationship between physical activity level, telomere length, and telomerase activity," *Med Sci Sports Exerc*, October 2008: 40(10):1764–71. doi: 10.1249/MSS.0b013e31817c92aa. PubMed PMID: 18799986; PubMed Central PMCID:PMC2581416.

27. S. A. Wolf, A. Melnik, and G. Kempermann. "Physical exercise increases adult neurogenesis and telomerase activity, and improves behavioral deficits in a mouse model of schizophrenia," *Brain Behav Immun*, July 2011: 25(5):971–80. doi: 10.1016/j.bbi.2010.10.014. Epub October 21, 2010. PubMed PMID: 20970493.

28. Lanza and Nair. "Mitochondrial function as a determinant of life span."

29. C. Werner, T. Fürster, T. Widmann, J. Pöss, C. Roggia, M. Hanhoun, J. Scharhag, N. Büchner, T. Meyer, W. Kindermann, J. Haendeler, M. Böhm, and U. Laufs. "Physical exercise prevents cellular senescence in circulating leukocytes and in the vessel wall," *Circulation*, December 15, 2009: 120(24):2438–47. doi: 10.1161/CIRCULATIONAHA.109.861005. Epub. PubMed PMID: 19948976.

30. Wroblewski et al. "Chronic exercise preserves lean muscle mass in masters athletes."

31. K. Meyer, R. Steiner, P. Lastayo, K. Lippuner, Y. Allemann, F. Eberli, J. Schmid, H. Saner, and H. Hoppeler. "Eccentric exercise in coronary patients: central hemodynamic and metabolic responses," *Med Sci Sports Exerc*, July 2003: 35(7):1076–82. PubMed PMID: 12840625.

32. J. K. Nelson and K. Zeratsky. "Do you have sitting disease?" July 25, 2012: http://www.mayoclinic.org/healthy-living/nutrition-and-healthy-eating/expert-blog/sitting-disease/bgp-20056238.

33. C. E. Matthews, K. Y. Chen, P. S. Freedson, M. S. Buchowski, B. M. Beech, R. R. Pate, and R. P. Troiano. "Amount of time spent in sedentary behaviors in the United States, 2003–2004," *Am J Epidemiol*, April 1, 2008: 167(7):875–81. doi: 10.1093/aje/kwm390. Epub February 25, 2008. PubMed PMID: 18303006; PubMed Central PMCID: PMC3527832.

34. H. M. Langevin. "Connective tissue: a body-wide signaling network?" *Med Hypotheses*, 2006; 66(6): 1074–7.

35. See: http://www.the-scientist.com/?articles.view/articleNo/35301/title/The-Science-of-Stretch.

36. Robert Schleip, "Fascia as a Sensory Organ" in *Dynamic Body Exploring Form, Expanding Function,* Erik Dalton and Judith Aston. (Oklahoma City: Freedom from Pain Institute, 2011), 137–163.

37. L. Berrueta, I. Muskaj, S. Olenich, T. Butler, G. J. Badger, R. A. Colas, M. Spite, C. N. Serhan, and H. M. Langevin. "Stretching Impacts Inflammation Resolution in Connective Tissue," *J Cell Physiol,* 2016;231(7): 1621–7.

38. Divo G. Müller and Robert Schleip: "Fascial Fitness—Suggestions for a fascia oriented training approach in sports and movement therapies": *Fascia: The Tensional Network of the Human Body,* ed. Robert Schleip, Thomas Findley, and Peter Huijing. (Edinburgh: Churchill Livingstone, 2009), 465–467.

39. Robert Schleip, Thomas Findley, Leon Chaitow, and Peter Huijing, ed., *Fascia: The Tensional Network of the Human Body* (Elsevier Health Sciences, 2013), 468.

40. N. T. Roach, M. Venkadesan, M. J. Rainbow, D. E. Lieberman. "Elastic energy storage in the shoulder and the evolution of high-speed throwing in Homo," *Nature.* 2013;498(7455): 483–6.

41. H. Langevin. "The effect of stretching on connective tissue: from tai chi to acupuncture," National Institutes of Health (NIH), *NIH Record,* November 23, 2012: 64(24), web.

42. M. A. Tarnopolsky. "Mitochondrial DNA shifting in older adults following resistance exercise training," *Appl Physiol Nutr Metab,* June 2009: 34(3):348–54. doi: 10.1139/H09–022. Review. PubMed PMID: 19448697.

43. M. Esmonde-White. *The Principles of Essentrics Program,* self-published, 2007.

44. H. Bronnum-Hansen, K. Juel, M. Davidsen, and J. Sorensen. "Impact of selected risk factors on expected lifetime without long-standing, limiting illness in Denmark," *Prev. Med* (2007): 45, 49–53.

45. Tarnopolsky. "ACSM Exchange Lecture: Exercise as a countermeasure for aging—from mice to humans."

46. C. Robb-Nicholson, MD. "The health benefits of tai chi," Harvard Medical School, Harvard Women's Health Watch, May 2009: www.health.harvard.edu.

47. G. Y. Yeh, MD, MPH; E. P. McCarthy, PhD; P. M. Wayne, PhD; L. W. Stevenson, MD; M. J. Wood, MD; D. Forman, MD; R. B. Davis, ScD; R. S. Phillips, MD. "Tai chi exercise in patients with chronic heart failure, a randomized clinical trial," *Journal of the American Medical Association, Arch Intern Med,* April 25, 2011: 171(8): 750–57, web.

48. K. Steib, I. Schäffner, R. Jagasia, B. Ebert, and D. C. Lie. "Mitochondria modify exercise-induced development of stem cell-derived neurons in the adult brain," *J Neurosci,* May 7, 2014: 34(19):6624–33. doi: 10.1523/JNEUROSCI.4972-13.2014. PubMed PMID: 24806687.

49. J. C. Smith, K. A. Nielson, J. L. Woodard, M. Seidenberg, S. Durgerian, K. E. Hazlett, C. M. Figueroa, C. C. Kandah, C. D. Kay, M. A. Matthews, and S. M. Rao. "Physical activity reduces hippocampal atrophy in elders at genetic risk for Alzheimer's disease," *Front Aging*

Neurosci, April 23, 2014: 6:61. doi: 10.3389/fnagi.2014.00061. eCollection 2014. PubMed PMID: 24795624; PubMed Central PMCID: PMC4005962.

50. J. A. Mortimer, D. Ding, A. R. Borenstein, C. DeCarli, Q. Guo, Y. Wu, Q. Zhao, and S. Chu. "Changes in brain volume and cognition in a randomized trial of exercise and social interaction in a community-based sample of non-demented Chinese elders," *Journal of Alzheimer's Disease*, IOS Press, March 26, 2012: 30(4).

51. Ibid.

52. Preamble to the Constitution of the World Health Organization as adopted by the International Health Conference, New York, June 19-22, 1946: signed on July 22, 1946 by the representatives of 61 states (Official Records of the World Health Organization, no. 2, p. 100) and entered into force on April 7, 1948.

53. Esmonde-White. *The Principles of Essentrics Program.*

54. M. Roig, K. Skriver, et al. "A single bout of exercise improves motor memory," *PLoS One.* 2012: 7(9): e44594. Published online September 4, 2012. doi: 10.1371/journal.pone.0044594 PMCID: PMC3433433.

INDEX

ABOUT THE AUTHOR

Miranda Esmonde-White is one of America's greatest advocates of and educators on healthy aging. She is best known for her PBS fitness show *Classical Stretch*, which has been on the air since 1999 with more than 300 episodes (many available on DVD). Miranda spent her childhood and teenage years studying at Canada's National Ballet School. Following her career as a professional ballerina, Miranda developed ESSENTRICS, the technique that Classical Stretch is based on. That work led to her becoming the flexibility trainer for numerous professional and Olympic athletes and celebrities: Medalist diver Alexandre Despatie, world squash champion Jonathon Power, Canadian skating champion Joannie Rochette, and students from the Cirque du Soleil School. In addition, her ESSENTRICS technique is used as the full-time stretch program by the Montreal Canadiens hockey team, actor Sarah Gadon, and supermodel Lily Cole. Miranda has also taught thousands of people in her worldwide ESSENTRICS classes, as well as a growing number of ESSENTRICS instructors in more than 20 countries. She travels throughout the world giving lectures, leading weeklong ESSENTRICS teacher training sessions, and facilitating restful retreats. In 2002, Miranda's daughter, Sahra, took over the marketing and management of Classical Stretch and ESSENTRICS. Through Sahra's marketing and management skills, ESSENTRICS became a world-renowned brand. The combined mother-daughter team has built ESSENTRICS into a respected international fitness company.

Find out more about Miranda and ESSENTRICS at

www.classicalstretch.com
www.essentrics.com
www.breastcancerrehabilitation.com